Scientific Writing
Easy when you know how

D0976583

Scientific Writing
Easy when you
know how

Jennifer Peat

Associate Professor, Department of Paediatrics and Child Health, University of Sydney and Hospital Statistician, The Children's Hospital at Westmead, Sydney, Australia

Elizabeth Elliott

Associate Professor, Department of Paediatrics and Child Health, University of Sydney and Consultant Paediatrician, The Children's Hospital at Westmead, Sydney, Australia

Louise Baur

Associate Professor, Department of Paediatrics and Child Health, University of Sydney and Consultant Paediatrician The Children's Hospital at Westmead, Sydney, Australia

Victoria Keena

Information Manager, Institute of Respiratory Medicine, Sydney, Australia

© BMJ Books 2002
BMJ Books is an imprint of the BMJ Publishing Group

First published in 2002
Second impression 2003
Third impression 2005
Fourth impression 2006
by BMJ Books, BMA House, Tavistock Square,
London WC1H 9JR

www.bmjbooks.com

British Library Cataloguing in Publication Data

A catalogue record for this book is available from the British Library

ISBN 13: 978 0 7279 1625 9
ISBN 10: 0 7279 1625 4

Typeset by SIVA Math Setters, Chennai, India
Printed and bound in Spain by GraphyCems, Navarra

Contents

Introduction

True ease in writing comes from art, not chance,
As those who move easiest have learnt to dance.

Alexander Pope (1688–1744)*

Everything is easy when you know how! The skill of scientific writing is no exception. To be a good writer, all you need to do is learn and then follow a few simple rules. However, it can be difficult to get a good grasp on the rules if your learning experience is a protracted process of trial and error. There is nothing more discouraging than handing a document that has taken hours to write to a coworker who takes a few minutes to cover it in red pen and expects you to find this a rewarding learning exercise.

Fortunately, there is a simple way into the more fulfilling experience of writing so that readers don't feel the need to suggest corrections for every sentence in every paragraph. Once you can write what you mean, put your content in the correct order, and make your document clear and pleasurable for others to read, you can consider yourself an expert writer. By developing good writing skills, you will receive more rewarding contributions from your coauthors and reviewers and more respect from the academic community. If you can produce a document that is well written, the review process automatically becomes a fulfilling contribution of academic ideas and thoughts rather than a desperate rescue attempt for bad grammar and disorganisation. This type of peer review is invaluable for improving the quality of your writing.

If your research is important for progressing scientific thinking or for improving health care, it deserves to be presented in the best possible way so that it will be published in a well-respected journal. This will ensure that your results reach a wide range of experts in your field. To use this process to promote your reputation, you will need to write clearly and concisely. Scientific writing is about using words correctly and

---

*The opening quote was produced with permission from *Collins Concise Dictionary of Quotations, 3rd edn*. London: Harper Collins, 1998: p 241.

finding a precise way to explain what you did, what you found, and why it matters. Your paper needs to be a clear recipe for your work:

- you need to construct an introduction that puts your work in context for your readers and tells them why it is important;
- your methods section must leave readers in no doubt what you did and must enable them to reproduce your work if they want to;
- you must present your results so that they can be easily understood, and discuss your findings so that readers appreciate the implications of your work.

In this book, we explain how to construct a framework for your scientific documents and for the paragraphs within so that your writing becomes orderly and structured. Throughout the book, we use the term "paper" to describe a document that is in the process of being written and the term "journal article" to describe a paper that has been published. At the end of some chapters, we have included lists of useful web sites and these are indicated by a reference in parenthesis (www[1]) in the text.

We also explain how the review and editorial process functions and we outline some of the basic rules of grammar and sentence construction. Although there is sometimes a relaxed attitude to grammar, it is important to have a few basic rules under your belt if you want to become a respected writer. To improve your professional status, it is best to be on high moral ground and write in a grammatically correct way so that your peers respect your work. You should not live in the hope that readers and editors will happily sort through muddled thoughts, struggle through verbose text, or tolerate an uninformed approach. Neither should you live in the hope that the journal and copy editors will rescue your worst grammatical mistakes. No one can guarantee that such safety systems will be in place and, to maintain quality and integrity in the research process, we should not expect other people to provide a final rescue system for poor writing.

The good news is that learning to write in a clear and correct way is easy. By following the guidelines presented in this book, the reporting of research results becomes a simple, rewarding process for many professional and personal reasons. We have tried not to be pedantic about what is right and what is wrong in pure linguistic or grammatical rules but rather to explain the rules that work best when presenting the results of scientific studies. We hope that novice writers will find this book of help to start them on a meaningful path to publishing their research, and that seasoned scientists will find some new tips to help them refine their writing skills.

Acknowledgements

We extend our thanks to the researchers who were noble enough to allow us to use their draft sentences in our examples. None of us writes perfectly to begin with or expects to see our first efforts displayed publicly. We are extremely grateful to the many people with whom we have worked and learnt from and we hope that they, in turn, receive satisfaction from helping others to become better writers.

Foreword

Editors need authors more than authors need editors. All authors and editors should remember this. Authors may be prone to despair and editors to arrogance, but authors are more important than editors. I was reminded of this eternal truth, which all editors forget, as I lectured yesterday in Calabar, Nigeria, on how to get published. I talked of the difficulty of writing and described the BMJ's system for triaging the 6000 studies submitted to us a year. It's nothing short of brutal. After the talk one of the audience asked: "What I want to know is what can you do for us?" Cheers went round the room.

All readers of this excellent book should remember their power over editors as they battle with the sometimes-difficult process of writing scientific papers. When the editor sends back a curt, incomprehensible, and unjustified rejection, you don't need necessarily to submit. Wise and experienced authors often will, sending their papers elsewhere and consoling themselves with the thought that the loss is to the journal not them. But if you feel like appealing, do. Don't explode into anger. Use the scalpel not the sword to refute the assertions of the editors and their reviewers. Perhaps they have said something sensible, in which case you might revise your paper accordingly. It's really the same technique that you should apply when stopped by the police. The result may well be acceptance.

Charged with the knowledge of your importance, I urge you to write. It can be a pleasure. Novelists describe how their characters take on lives of their own, beginning to amaze and fascinate their creators. Something similar can happen with scientific papers. As you write you may think new – and sometimes exciting – thoughts. Certainly you will be forced to clarify your thoughts. If you can't write it clearly then you probably haven't thought it clearly. As you wrestle with the words new insights should occur. What you didn't understand you will have to understand. I probably shouldn't admit this, but I never quite know what I think until I write it down. The same goes for my speaking, which causes me much more trouble: what's written can and should be edited, whereas what's said cannot be withdrawn.

The broad messages I try to deliver when talking on how to get published are the same as those in this book. The first reason to write is because you have something important to say. Ideally you will want to describe a stunning piece of research. You will have a valid answer to an important scientific or clinical question that nobody has answered before. If you have such a treasure, then you would need to be a worse author than McGonigle was poet in order to fail to achieve publication. Only if you achieve the opacity of London smog will we fail to discern the importance of your research.

Once you have something to say you need a structure for your paper. This, I believe, is the most important part of writing. There is nothing more awful for readers to be lost in a sea of words, unsure where they came from, where they are, and where they are headed. They will stop reading and move on to something more interesting. "Remember" I tell authors, "you compete with Manchester United, Hollywood films, and the world's greatest writers. A very few people may have to read your paper (perhaps you supervisor), but most won't. You are part of 'the attention economy' and competing for peoples' attention."

There are many structures. At school you were probably taught to have "a beginning, a middle, and an end." Unfortunately, this usually becomes what the poet Philip Larkin called "a beginning, a muddle, and an end." You might try a sonnet, a limerick, or a haiku (in our 2001Christmas issue of the BMJ we published a haiku version of every scientific study), but both you and your readers probably want something easier. Another English poet, Rudyard Kipling, described the structure used by most reporters:

I keep six honest serving men
(They taught me all I know),
Their names are What and Why and When,
And How and Where and Who?

If a bomb goes off, reporters want answers to all those questions.

And these questions are the basis for the famous IMRaD (Introduction, Methods, Results, and Discussion) structure of scientific papers. The introduction says why you did the study, the methods describe what you did and the results what you found, and the discussion (the most difficult part of the paper by far) the implications of your findings.

The beauty of the IMRaD structure is not only that it is ready made for you but also that it is familiar to your readers. They won't be lost. Even if it's unconscious they know their way around a paper written in the IMRaD structure. Peter Medawar, a great scientist and writer, was scornful of the IMRaD structure, arguing correctly that it doesn't reflect how science happens. The doing of science is much messier. If you can write as well as Medawar then you can safely ignore the IMRaD structure, but almost none of us can – which is why we should pay homage to and use the IMRaD structure.

Once you have your structure you must spin your words, and here, as every expert on style agrees, you should keep it as simple as possible. Use short words and short paragraphs, always prefer the simple to the complex, and stick to nouns and verbs (the bone and muscle of writing). "Good prose," said George Orwell, "is like a window pane." Mathew Arnold defined "the essence of style" as "having something to say and saying it as clearly as you can." I suggest that you take a child rather than Henry James as your model. There is a place for highly wrought, beautiful writing, but it isn't in a scientific paper – and most of us can't do it anyway.

Most of us can't write like James, Hemingway, or Proust, but all of us should, with help, be able to write a scientific paper. This excellent book provides that help.

Richard Smith
Editor, BMJ

Competing interest: Richard Smith is the chief executive of the BMJ Publishing Group, which is publishing this book. He is, however, paid a fixed salary and will not benefit financially even if this book sells as many copies as a Harry Potter book. He wasn't even paid to write this introduction, illustrating Johnson's maxim that "only a fool would write for any reason apart from money."

1: Scientific writing

What is written without effort is in general read without pleasure.

Samuel Johnson (1709–1784)

The objectives of this chapter are to understand:

- the importance of publishing research results
- how to organise your time to write a paper
- the components of writing that make up a paper

Reasons to publish

Scientists communicate the fruits of their labour mostly in writing, and mostly in scientific journals. Conferences and other forms of verbal communication, including the evening news, play an important role but the written word reaches the widest audience and constitutes the archival message.

Kenneth Rothman (www[1])

It is important to publish research results for many reasons. In the most basic sense, it is unethical to enrol participants in a research study with their understanding that you will answer an important research question and then fail to report the study results in a timely manner. It is also unethical to accept a grant from a funding body and then fail to publish the results of the research that you conducted using the funds. Failure to publish reflects badly on your reputation as a scientist and is likely to have a significant influence on your future career and your ability to attract further funding. On the other hand, success in publishing contributes to rewards such as job promotion and professional recognition.

A scientific article that is published in a well-respected, peer-reviewed journal is an important goal for any researcher and remains one of the ultimate markers of research success. For this reason, it is important to write your paper well so that it has clear messages, is readily accepted for publication, and is something that you can always be proud of.

A well-written paper is one that is easy to read, tells an interesting story, has the information under the correct headings, and is visually appealing. It is a sad fact of life that few researchers or clinicians read a journal article from beginning to end. Most readers want to scan your paper quickly and find the relevant information where they expect it to be. If you want the information in your paper to be read and to be used, you must be certain that you have presented it in an organised and accessible format.

In the current academic climate, publications are imperative for career advancement and for the economic survival of research departments. In many institutions, the number of successful publications is used as a measure of research productivity. In addition, other attributes of publications, such as the number of collaborators, the number of resulting citations, and the impact factor of the journal, are often considered. As such, publications are a fundamental marker of accountability. Box 1.1 summarises some of the important reasons for publishing your work.

Box 1.1 Reasons to publish your research results

It is unethical to conduct a study and not report the findings
You have some results that are worth reporting
You want to progress scientific thought or improve health outcomes
You want to give credibility to your research team
You want your work to reach a broad audience
Your track record will improve
You will add credibility to your reputation
You will improve your chance of promotion
You are more likely to obtain research grants

Motives to publish vary widely. Some researchers may have a driving force to contribute to advancements in scientific knowledge and improvements in patient care, or may simply love their work and want to share it with others. Other researchers may work in a unit that has a "publish or perish" imperative so that journal articles are essential for professional survival. Whatever your motive, you will need something important to say if you want your results to be published. A report of the sixtieth case of a rare condition is unlikely to be published even if it makes fascinating reading. Similarly, reports of uncontrolled clinical studies, inadequately evaluated interventions, or laboratory data that do not address the underlying mechanisms of a disease are unlikely to be published in a good journal. To improve your chances of being published, your study must have a rigorous design, your results must answer an important question, and your paper must be written well. A well-designed and well-reported study is always a good candidate for being accepted by a respected journal.

Rewards for being a good writer

Generally keep it short and to the point. It is not a novel you are writing. If you get stuck, take a break. Leave the draft by your bedside. Sometimes a phrase just comes to you and it is a shame to lose it.

Anthony David[1]

Having good scientific writing skills can not only bring career success but also brings many other personal rewards as shown in Box 1.2. These rewards are often fundamental for job promotion in a world in which grant applications, published journal articles, and oral presentations are used as formal indicators of research performance. These indicators may also be critical at a departmental level where the number of successful grant applications, postgraduate students, and publications are used as formal markers of team productivity.

Box 1.2 Reasons to be a good writer

Writing time is more productive and less frustrating
Peers will take you more seriously
Your research is more likely to lead to publications
Your grant applications are more likely to be funded
Your expertise will help you to become a good reviewer or editor

---

A well-written paper is one that is very publishable, adds credibility to your reputation, and is much more likely to be read in its entirety and thus taken seriously by the scientific community. Bad science is not usually publishable (although it happens) but good science reported well is more highly respected than good science reported badly. Of course, mind-blowing discoveries will always be respected no matter how they are written. Few of us are lucky enough to have such discoveries to report but even exciting new findings are better appreciated if they are written elegantly. The famous phrase "It has not escaped our notice that ..." from Watson and Crick when they reported their discovery of the double helix[2] is a prime example. The sentence that they wrote was *It has not escaped our notice that the specific pairing we have postulated immediately suggests a possible copying mechanism for the genetic material.* This was a modest way to declare that they had discovered a structure for DNA that was both biologically feasible and would facilitate the replication of genetic material. The article was a model in concise writing in that it occupied only one page of *Nature*.

Most researchers will never be able to emulate the importance of the findings of Watson and Crick, although we may strive to emulate their concise writing style.

There is no doubt that good writing skills will bring you a more rewarding research career because fewer keyboard hours will need to be spent on each published paper. Long hours spent at the computer rearranging pages of print are not the best way to achieving a happy and healthy life. By reducing the time it takes from first draft to final product, good writing skills are a passport to both academic success and personal fulfilment.

In being a good writer, you will automatically become a good reviewer. By definition, reviewers are experts in their field who are asked to assess the scientific validity of submitted papers or grant applications. Being an experienced reviewer also leads to invitations to participate in advisory bodies that make decisions about the scientific merit of proposed studies, that judge posters or presentations at scientific meetings, or that have the responsibility of marking a postgraduate thesis. All of these positions are rewarding recognition that you have that certain talent that has an important currency in the scientific community.

Making it happen

> *"Do it every day for a while" my father kept saying. "Do it as you would do scales on the piano. Do it by pre-arrangement with yourself. Do it as a debt of honour. And make a commitment to finishing things."*
>
> Anne Lamott[3]

Scientific documents cannot happen unless they are given priority in life. To achieve this, it is important to develop good time management skills that enable you to distinguish between the urgent and the important issues in your working day.[4] Before you begin writing, you need to get on top of the urgent and important tasks for the day. It's a matter of addressing the crises, completing the deadlines, and getting the pressing matters off your desk and out of your mind. It is also a good idea to be aware of, and minimise, the urgent but unimportant matters such as unnecessary mail and meetings that tend to waste the day away. If you let the unimportant matters fill up your day, you will never find enough time to write.

Committed researchers need the skills to programme dedicated writing time into their working week. In an excellent book on time management, the focus on important tasks is described as spending time on "quadrant II activity".[4] An adaptation of the quadrants in which you can spend time is shown in Table 1.1. By definition, quadrant II activities are not urgent but they have to be acted upon because they are important to career success. By minimising the amount of time you spend on the urgent and important activities in quadrant I and by avoiding non-important activities in quadrants III and IV, you can spend more time on prime writing and thereby become more productive. It is prudent to remember that there is no such thing as having no time to write. We all have 24 hours each day and it is up to each of us to decide how we allocate this time.

If you are serious about wanting to publish your work, you need to schedule adequate time for the activity of writing in the "important but non-urgent" quadrant. There is good evidence that this works. By rising at 5am every morning and writing for several hours every day, Anthony Trollope completed more than fifty books and became one of England's

Table 1.1 Time management[4].

	Urgent	Not urgent
Important	**Quadrant I** Crises, deadlines, patient care, teaching, some meetings, preparation	**Quadrant II** Research, writing, reading, professional development, physical health, and family
Not important	**Quadrant III** Some phone calls, emails, mail, meetings, and popular activities, for example morning and afternoon teas	**Quadrant IV** Junk mail, some phone calls and emails, time wasters, and escape activities, for example internet browsing, playing computer games, reading magazines, watching TV

most renowned 19th century novelists. Although many of us would argue that Jane Austen or Thomas Hardy wrote much more interesting novels, no one can doubt that Trollope's commitment to his writing and his time management skills led to greater productivity.

When you are researching, scheduling time for quadrant II activities ensures that you can give priority to designing the study, collecting the data, analysing the results, and writing the papers. Many researchers have no problem finding time to conduct the study but have difficulty in finding time for writing. The good news is that constructing a paper will be more rewarding if you develop good writing skills and you will come to enjoy using your "quadrant II" activity time more effectively.

Once your data analyses are underway and the aims of the paper are decided, you should begin writing in earnest. Ideally, you will have presented your results at departmental meetings, at local research meetings, or even at a national or international conference. This will have helped you to refine your ideas about how to interpret your data. You may also have a feel for the topics that need to be addressed in the discussion. With all this behind you and with good writing skills, putting the paper together should be a piece of cake.

Achieving creativity

You should allow yourself to get into a writing mood. Finish the background reading, the review of the literature, and the work to date. You know it inside out. Relax. Take deep breaths. Just let it flow. Many people find music a help but choose carefullly ... Wear comfortable clothes; a sweater and jeans are fine.

Anthony David[1]

To write effectively, you need to find a physical space where you can both work and think. This space is probably not going to be the same office from which you conduct consultations, direct staff, take phone calls and answer endless emails and voicemails in the course of everyday business. For most people, a clear, thinking space needs to be a place where interruptions are minimal and so, by necessity, will be away from your daily work environment.

Your thinking space needs to be a place where you can feel comfortable and relaxed, where you don't have to power dress if you don't want to, and where you can play thinking music if you find that helps you to write.[1] "Mufti" days were invented so that people could relax in the freedom of not having to wear their working uniform. If it helps, award yourself a mufti day and choose some appropriate music. For some people baroque or flute music is ideal, for others Mark Knoffler or Red Hot Chilli Peppers does the job perfectly. Italian opera is definitely too dramatic and blues or jazz may leave you focused on some of the sadder events in life. You need music that will relax but not distract you – the choice is entirely up to you.

To write effectively, you must also tune in to your creative day and your creative hour. For some people, Thursdays, Fridays, and Saturdays are best because most of the urgent processes of the week are over. Others may find the pending excitement of the weekend distracting and thus prefer to begin writing refreshed on a Monday. Some people who are morning writers can happily word process their ideas whilst ignoring everything around them that will wait until later in the day when their creativity has burnt out. Others may be afternoon writers who need to deal with the quadrant I matters first and work up to writing when the urgent list is clear. It doesn't matter when or where you write, as long as you choose your best opportunities and organise yourself accordingly.

Whatever your creativity pattern, it is important to visit your writing as often as possible, every day if you can. Writing new text may take a significant amount of work but reading and reviewing written text to polish it up can often fit into short time blocks and can be done anywhere. When you have spare moments to edit your writing, you need to inspect your sentences and your paragraphs for needless words, silly flaws, and clumsy transitions. Writing is a process of constant repair but if you are passionate about your research this will not be arduous. It will be exciting to see your paper taking shape, becoming simple and clear, and acquiring impact. Refining your writing so that it takes on more form and character and becomes easy to read is well worthwhile. This is one of the hallmarks of scientific writing.

Thought, structure, and style

And whenever I see a first novel dedicated to a wife (or a husband), I smile and think "There's someone who knows". Writing is a lonely job. Having someone who believes in you makes a lot of difference. They don't have to make speeches. Just believing is enough.

Stephen King[5]

Scientific writing is a well-defined technique rather than a creative art. The three basic aspects to effective scientific writing are thought, structure, and style.

- *Thought* is a matter of having some worthwhile results and ideas to publish. You need some new results to publish and you need to be able to interpret them correctly.

- *Structure* is simply a matter of getting the right things in the right place.
- *Style* is a matter of choosing the fewest and most appropriate words and using the rules of good grammar.

When you ask for feedback on the thoughts and structure of your paper, you are asking for a macro-review of the basic content. On the other hand, if you ask for feedback on the style you are asking for a micro-review of the words, grammar, and order. In a sense, there is little point in a reviewer providing feedback on the style until the thoughts and structure are in place. To gain the most from peer review, you should be clear about the type of feedback you would appreciate most and whether your paper is sufficiently advanced to ask for micro-feedback.

Constructing a well-organised paper is the first step to improving accessibility and readability. A nicely structured paper with no worthwhile results, or worthwhile results in a badly structured paper, are unlikely to be published. Moreover, papers that are written in a poor style in terms of expression and grammar are unlikely to appeal to editors, reviewers, or fellow scientists, and are also unlikely to be published in a good journal. In Chapters 2 and 3, we explain how to present your thoughts and academic ideas using the correct structure, and in Chapters 8–11 we give examples of how to write in a clear style. The web site resources that may be of help are listed at the end of each chapter and are referenced as (www[1]) throughout. All website addresses were current when this book went to press.

The thrill of acceptance

Seeing your name in print is such an amazing concept: you get so much attention without having to actually show up somewhere... There are many obvious advantages to this. You don't have to dress up, for instance, and you can't hear them boo you straight away.

Anne Lamott[3]

There are relatively few high points in research but most of us recognise one when we see one. Some high points that spring to mind are the acceptance of a paper by a journal, conducting a data analysis that confirms your hypothesis, and news that a grant application has been successful. Certainly, having a paper accepted is one of the most far-reaching successes. The corollary is that having a paper rejected is a depressing and crushing event that is worth trying to avoid.

After a paper has been sent to a journal, there is always a time of apprehension while you wait for a reply. This can take from weeks if you are lucky, to months if you are not. For some journals, electronic submission and electronic communication with external reviewers has expedited the review process. Whether electronic or manual, the first letter that returns from the journal generally confirms the arrival of your paper on the editorial desk. The next letter is much more fundamental in that it is likely to signal acceptance or rejection. This letter always brings a frisson of terror and expectation as you open it, and then either elation or devastation when you read it. It's never any different. All papers are important to their authors and there is no middle ground between potential acceptance and outright rejection. If you ever have difficulty in writing, it may be encouraging to think of the thrill of the moment when your paper is accepted for publication. It is a heady moment, one of the true highs in research and an event that is worth striving towards.

Acknowledgements

King quotes have been reprinted with the permission of Scribner, a Division of Simon & Schuster, Inc., from *On Writing: A Memoir of the Craft* by Stephen King. Copyright © by Stephen King. The Johnson quote has been produced with permission from *Collins Concise Dictionary of Quotations, 3rd edn*. London: Harper Collins, 1998 (p 175). All other referenced quotes have been produced with permission.

Websites

1 Rothman K. Writing for epidemiology. *Epidemiology* 1998;9. www.epidem. com

References

1 David A. Write a classic paper. *BMJ* 1990;**300**:30–1.
2 Watson JD, Crick FHC. Molecular structure of nucleic acids. A structure for deoxyribose nucleic acid. *Nature* 1953;**171**:737–8.
3 Lamott A. *Some instructions on writing and life*. Peterborough: Anchor Books, 1994; p xi–xxxi.
4 Covey SR, Merrill AR, Merrill RR. The urgency addiction. In: *First things first*. London: Simon and Schuster, 1994; p 32–43.
5 King S. *On writing: A memoir of the craft*. London: Scribner, 2000; p 74.

2: Getting started

Scientists who become authors display a rich variety of publication habits. Isaac Newton was famously reluctant to publish and, when he did, to put his name to the work. More recently, and less famously, Yury Struchkov published one paper every 3.9 days for 10 years, while 20 researchers worldwide each published at least once every 11.3 days throughout the decade of the 1980s.

Drummond Rennie[1]

The objectives of this chapter are to understand how to:

- plan your paper
- choose an appropriate journal
- prepare your paper in the correct format
- make decisions about authorship
- decide who is a contributor and who should be acknowledged

Journal articles form the most important part of a researcher's bibliography because they publish the results of their original research. To be published, your paper must be constructed in the approved manner and presented to the highest possible standards.[2] If your research is important, then you should plan for your results to reach the widest possible audience. This means constructing your paper well, writing it nicely, and having it accepted in a widely read peer-reviewed journal. Most of this book is dedicated to writing and publishing a journal article. The methods for constructing a paper are discussed in Chapters 3 and 4, and the methods for publishing your paper are discussed in Chapters 5 and 6.

Forming a plan

I want to suggest that to write to your best abilities, it behooves you to construct your own toolbox and then build up enough muscle so you can carry it with you. Then, instead of looking at a hard job and getting discouraged, you will perhaps seize the correct tool and get immediately to work.

Stephen King[3]

Constructing a paper is easy if you begin with a plan in mind. By using a template to put your paper together and by assembling your thoughts in a logical order, the task becomes much less daunting than you might imagine. You also need to follow some simple rules when planning and writing your paragraphs and then your sentences. It is important that papers are not allowed to meander and grow in an unplanned way. If you were building a house or having a special dinner party, you would work to a plan, so why not do this with something that is as fundamental to your research career as a scientific publication? This chapter will explain how writing using a logical framework helps you to structure your paper correctly, which then helps to prevent your readers and reviewers from getting lost. Once your paper has a logical structure, Chapters 8–11 will help you to improve your writing style.

Throughout the writing process, you must focus on the potential audience for whom you are writing your paper. The editor and external peer reviewers of a journal are the only people whom you have to impress in order to get your work into print, so write explicitly for them. Odds on, if these people think that your work is worth publishing, then the scientific audience that you hope to reach will think so too. If you are writing a postgraduate thesis, then plan to write to impress your examiners. Your examiners may be the only people who ever read your thesis in its entirety, and they have a major influence on whether you receive your degree.

Most writers have access to a computer with word processing software that can speed up the process of writing considerably. However, without proper document planning, the facility to "cut and paste" can often lead to unnecessary and unproductive shuffling of text. Creating a sound structure from the outset can help to avoid this. This makes the writing process more purposeful and circumvents the frustration of having to live through just one or two drafts too many. Some writers still prefer to write by hand, especially in the planning stages of a paper. If you prefer this, then document planning is especially important for you.

If you are using a computer to write your paper, then it is important that you use all of the software facilities that you have at your disposal. Headers and footers can be used to label your paper, number the pages and date the draft on which you are working. Your software can also be used to create standard formats for the major headings, subheadings, and minor headings throughout the document. Your page facility will enable you to set your margins so that they are correct for the journal, and tools such as spell check and word count are invaluable. The efficient use of these tools is both professional and efficient in terms of time management.

Before your fingers even think about approaching the keyboard or picking up a pen, you should have conferred with your authorship team about the specific questions that you will answer in your paper. In an ideal world, you would also have decided to which journal you are going to submit your work and you will have obtained their "Instructions to authors". Then you can begin.

First, you will need to start the document by inserting the headings and subheadings that you will be using. By forming a framework into which to assemble your aims, your methods, your findings, and your thoughts, you will find that all of your material falls into the correct places. Figure 2.1 shows a plan for putting a paper together and progressing your paper from the initial planning stages to the final document.

In starting your first draft, a divide and conquer approach is best. The best thing about a grotty first draft is that it is a great starting point, giving you something to build later drafts on. In most journals, reporting is usually confined to the IMRAD (introduction, methods, results, and discussion) format, so begin by putting "Introduction" at the top of one page, "Methods" at the top of the next, "Results" at the top of the next, and so on. Next, you begin to fill each section in. Just do one bit at a time starting with the simplest parts such as the methods and the results. Then you have begun.

Approach each section with its length and content in mind. A paper should be no longer than 2000–2500 words, which will occupy only 8–10 double-spaced pages in draft copy. Some journals set limits such as four or six pages for the final published copy, including the tables and figures. Table 2.1 shows the amount of space that each section of an average draft paper should occupy. Do not plan to write more than

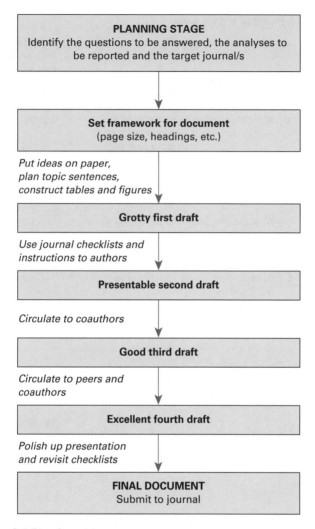

Figure 2.1 Plan for writing a paper.

this. All journals differ in their requirements but few papers are rejected because they are too short.

Remember that it is neither efficient nor satisfying to write everything you know in 30 or 40 pages, and then have to prune and reorganise it yourself, or ask your reviewers to do this for you. Although this approach may foster creativity and

Table 2.1 Planning a draft paper.

Section	Question to be answered	Purpose	Expected length with A4 paper, font size 10–12 and 1·5 line spacing
Introduction	Why did you start?	Summarise the context of your study and state the aims clearly	1 page
Methods	What did you do?	Give enough detail for the study to be repeated	2–3 pages
Results	What did you find?	Describe the study sample and use the data analyses to answer the aims	2–3 pages
Tables and figures	What do the results show?	Clarify the results	3–6 tables or figures
Discussion	What does it mean?	Interpret your findings in context of other literature and describe their potential impact on health care	2–3 pages
References	Who else has done important work in your field?	Cite the most relevant and most recent literature	20–35 references
Total document			**12–20 pages**

lateral thinking, it is not helpful for the expedient reporting of your results or for the efficient use of your own and your peer reviewers' time. Keep in mind that your purpose in writing a scientific paper is to answer a specific research question or fulfil a specific research aim. You should provide only sufficient background about why you did the study, sufficient methods to repeat the study, and sufficient data and explanations to understand the results. Do not be tempted to deviate from this path. Readers do not need to know absolutely everything that you know about the research area.

Scientific writing is not a competition in comprehensiveness. You must limit yourself to writing only the essential information that your readers need to know about the results that you are reporting.

You will need to progress your paper from your grotty first draft to a presentable second draft before you start asking coauthors and coworkers for peer review. There are many checklists available, including checklists for critical appraisal, that are a good guide to the information that you will need to include in each section of your paper.[4-7] The *BMJ* also has excellent checklists for writers, reviewers and statisticians that can be accessed through its web site (www[1]). Progressing through each draft may take many small rewrites and reorganisations of sentences and paragraphs but it will ensure that the feedback you get is worth having. Once you have a presentable second draft you can sequentially ask for peer review from wider sources to improve your paper. In Chapter 4, we discuss how to manage the peer-review process effectively.

Choosing a journal

Will your message appeal to your reader? Will it be read? I cannot overstate the importance of this invisible bridge. Many important, even vital, messages are lost in the inappropriate translation from author to reader. Above all else, write for your intended reader; all that follows stems from this rapport.

Vincent Fulginiti[8]

Once you have planned your paper, you will need to choose a journal in which to publish it. This can be a complex decision. Over 4500 journals in 30 languages are currently listed in *Index Medicus* (www[2]) and more than 150 scientific journal articles are published each day. Despite these daunting statistics, it is always best to write with a specific journal in mind. The first question to ask yourself is what type of audience you want to reach. It is important to make an initial decision about whether you want to publish in a general, clinical, or speciality journal, or in a journal that publishes the results of basic science. For example, the journal *Diabetes Care* publishes papers about the diagnosis and treatment of diabetic patients, whereas the journal *Diabetes* also publishes articles that report the results of bench-top research.

You also need to decide whether you want to publish in a relatively new journal or in a well-established journal, and in a journal that comes out weekly, monthly, or quarterly. Finally, you need to have a good idea about whether your results will be more relevant to an international or local audience. Your choice of journal will be influenced by your subject matter and will, in turn, also influence the audience that your work reaches. The journal that you choose will have important implications for the time that it takes for your paper to be published, the impact that it will have, and the prestige that it will bring back to you.

New journals may be more likely to accept papers but often have low impact factors (see Chapter 6), may have limited circulation, and may not reach a wide audience. On the other hand, highly ranked established journals are harder to get into and may have long wait times between article acceptance and publication. Established journals with a high profile are much more likely to be read by people who are experts in your field, and they carry inestimable prestige. If you submit your paper to an established journal, it may be rejected, but you may reap unexpected gains in that you will receive pertinent reviews that enable you to improve your reporting.

Acceptance rates vary widely. Established journals that are committed to short publication times may accept only a small percentage of submitted papers. The *BMJ* publishes only 14–17% of over 4000 papers submitted each year[9] and *JAMA* published only 11% of the 4366 manuscripts submitted.[10,11] Other journals accept about one third of papers.[12] Up to 50% of papers may be rejected at the editorial review and many others that elicit a positive review from external reviewers do not go on to publication. Most journals publish only between 10–50% of papers. With rejection rates running high, having an important message to report and reporting it well is essential for increasing your chance of being published.

There is a delicate balance between aiming high, trying to maximise the possibility of acceptance, and trying to reduce the time to publication. Some useful considerations when deciding where to publish are shown in Box 2.1. In deciding which journal to select, seek advice widely from your coauthors and peers, but be aware that their advice will be subjective and that their agenda may be very different from your own. It is a good idea to choose three or four journals in which you are most interested and rank them in order of prestige and competitiveness. This may help you to decide whether you want to send your paper to a highly regarded journal where you may be rejected but which will bring inestimable prestige if accepted. Alternatively, you may want to send your paper to a journal where you stand a good chance of being accepted or to a journal where acceptance is most likely. One thing is certain – you will never be published in a prestigious journal if you never submit your work there.

Box 2.1 Deciding where to submit

Use corporate experience
Match your paper with the personality and scope of the journal
Match your subject with the journal's target audience
Consider the impact factor and citation index of the journal
Weigh up the journal prestige, the likelihood of acceptance and the
    likely time until publication
Have realistic expectations
Scan the journals for one that matches your content and study
    design
Be robust and, if rejected, select another journal

To ensure that your paper is published, it helps to have research results that are new, that are important, and that are relevant to your potential readership. In this, the journal you choose will need to be well suited to your research findings, and the topic of your paper will need to fall within the scope of the journal. For example, the results of a large randomised controlled trial of an innovative and effective treatment for breast cancer may be best submitted to the *New England Journal of Medicine*. However, details of a newly identified gene may be best submitted to *Nature Genetics*, and an epidemiological study to assess the prevalence of a childhood illness may be best submitted to the *Archives of Diseases in Childhood*. The concept that negative results are harder to place than positive results is supported by documented publication bias.[13–15] The time to publication is often delayed for studies that report negative findings or non-significant results. Classic examples of this are the delayed publication of negative results from randomised controlled trials[16] and for studies that have reported non-significant health effects of passive smoking.[17]

Remember that if you are writing for a general journal then you cannot use the same language as that for a specialist journal. However, regardless of the journal, your writing must always be easy to understand by both the external reviewers and the audience that you expect to reach. If your message is important, then delivering it in an entirely effective way will help to disseminate your results to the research and medical community where they really matter. On the other hand, if you don't have an important question, good data with which to answer it, and a clear message for your audience, you should think twice about starting to write the paper.

You should try to reach a consensus with your coauthors about preferred journals when you are first ready to start writing your paper. This will help you to decide on the style and the format in which you will write and, in turn, save you from the frustration and time that it takes to change your paper and the format of your citations from one journal to another. Since different journals require you to present your text and/or analyses in different formats, the earlier you make the decision about the journal the sooner you can begin formatting your paper in the correct style. Some journals resist figures and prefer tables, some journals resist the use of percentages and prefer you to give both the numerators and denominators in the tables, and some journals have a limit on the number of tables, figures, or citations that they will accept. Some journals request that you check your spelling using the *Oxford English Dictionary*, others specify the *Macquarie Dictionary* or *Webster's Dictionary*. It is best to know about the quirks of your journal of first choice so that you can adopt their format early in the piece.

To expedite the publication of your work, try to be realistic and choose the right journal first time. However, if your paper is rejected and you decide to submit it to a second journal, then keep in mind that some journals request that you also send the previous reviewers' comments plus your responses. The editor will want to be assured that you have addressed and/or amended any problems that have already been identified. There are no published statistics about journal shopping practices, but an editor will obviously not be interested in a paper that has been rejected from other journals on the basis of fundamental problems with study design. Remember that if you do submit to another journal, reading the instructions to authors and modifying the manuscript accordingly will improve your chances of publication. This may also save you time because many journals will automatically return papers that do not meet their standards.

A study by researchers at Stanford University suggested that prestige, whether the journal usually publishes papers on a particular topic, and reader profiles are important factors that influence decisions about where to send a manuscript.[18] However, other more pragmatic factors, such as likelihood of acceptance, turnaround time, circulation size, previous publications, and recommendations of colleagues are often considered. In the end, your decision on where to send your paper will be based on many factors and, in deciding, you will need to respect the advice of your colleagues and coauthors.

Uniform requirements

The Uniform Requirements are instructions to authors on how to prepare manuscripts, not to editors on publication style.

International Committee of Medical Journal editors (www[3])

All draft papers should be prepared in a format that is consistent with the "Uniform requirements for manuscripts submitted to biomedical journals".[19] These requirements were first developed in 1978 when a group of journal editors met in Vancouver to establish guidelines for the format of manuscripts submitted to their journals. The group naturally became known as the Vancouver group and the standard format is still referred to as Vancouver format. The first uniform requirements for manuscripts and recommendations for formatting references were published in 1979, and an updated version can now be accessed via the world wide web (www[3]).

The Vancouver group eventually evolved into the International Council of Medical Journal Editors (ICMJE) who publish the uniform requirements on their website. The ICMJE uniform requirements have been revised at intervals since their inception and are now widely adopted by the majority of medical journals. If you are writing a scientific paper, you need to be conversant with these standardised requirements for formatting both your paper and your reference list. Although some journals still have significantly different format requirements for references, the advent of reference database software (www[4]) means that lists can be more easily changed to different formats.

Over 500 journals now use the ICMJE uniform requirements and either cite the document or make reference to it in their instructions to authors. The uniform requirements are clear and concise instructions to authors on how to prepare a manuscript for submission to a journal and which style to adopt. Some examples of the uniform requirements are shown in Box 2.2. In the event of the acceptance of your paper for publication, the copy editor may ultimately change your style. However, regardless of publication style, many journals still require papers to be submitted according to the standard uniform requirements.

Box 2.2 Examples of some of the uniform requirements for manuscripts[19]

Use double spacing throughout

Pages should have margins at least 25 mm and be numbered

Maintain the sequence title page, abstract, key words, text, acknowledgements, references, tables, legends to figures

The title page should carry the title, a short running title, information of any disclaimers or funding bodies and the authors' full names, qualifications, affiliations, departments, and addresses

Text should be presented under the headings Introduction, Methods, Results, and Discussion

Begin each section on a new page

Each table should be on a new page

Illustrations and unmounted prints should be labelled on the back with the author's name and the figure number, and should be no larger than 203 × 254 mm

Include permission to reproduce previously published material or to use illustrations that may identify participants

Enclose a transfer of copyright

Submit the required number of paper copies

Enclose an electronic copy if required—the disk should have the author's name, file name, and format labelled clearly

Keep an exact copy of everything submitted

Instructions to authors

A basic rule is to read the instructions to authors. Too few authors do this, but there is little point in writing a 400 word introduction when the journal has a limit for the whole article of 600 words.

Richard Smith[20]

Although many journals require papers to be submitted according to the uniform requirements, each journal also has its own instructions to authors that are published on the journal website or in the printed copy of the journal. Sometimes the instructions are only published once or twice a year, for example, *JAMA* publishes its instructions to authors in January and July. The instructions to authors for many journals can be accessed via a central Medical College of Ohio website (www[5]). As soon as you have decided where to submit your paper, you should obtain the instructions to authors, read them carefully, make note of all of the relevant points, and then read them carefully again. In addition to requiring papers to conform to the uniform requirements, each journal often lists its own specific submission requirements. These may include the number of copies of the paper to submit, use of abbreviations, the standard dictionary to be used for spelling, the maximum length of the paper, the style for references, and so on.

Any time you spend on formatting before you submit your paper to a journal is time well spent. If your paper conforms exactly to a journal's guidelines, it is much more likely to be received favourably by the editor. This will help to ensure that your paper is processed expeditiously and that unnecessary delays are avoided. If you do not follow the guidelines, your manuscript may be returned to you before it is sent out for external peer review, thus causing unnecessary delay and wasting precious time.

Most papers can be shortened without detracting from their impact. Some journals have a policy of returning papers that exceed the established length limits and ask authors to shorten them before they are sent out for review. Even when papers that exceed page limits are sent out for peer review, they may ultimately be rejected solely on the basis of their length and despite the scientific merit of the content. Shortening a paper so that it conforms to the limits set by a journal should not be too onerous. If you are having problems with word-trimming, consider whether each table needs all the information it shows, whether you have duplicated any of the information in the text and whether all of the tables and figures are absolutely essential for conveying your main results. If you have presented the same results as both categorical and continuous data analyses, one of the two approaches could probably be omitted. It is also worth considering whether all of the information in the introduction and discussion is essential for putting your work in the context of the literature. By cutting out words, sentences, and paragraphs here and there, it is always possible to reduce the length of a paper without compromising the main messages. Some ways to do this are discussed in Chapter 8. If you are too emotionally involved with your writing to be objective about making cuts, it is probably best to enrol someone else to help you do it.

Standardised reporting guidelines

Writing is the only thing that, when I do it, I don't feel I should be doing something else.

Gloria Steinem (www.bartelby.com)

Standardised guidelines for reporting certain types of studies have been developed and go under acronyms such as CONSORT, MOOSE, QUOROM, and STARD, as explained below. The Consolidated Standards of Reporting Trials (CONSORT) guidelines were developed by an expert group of researchers, epidemiologists, journal editors, and statisticians (www[6]). The ICMJE recommends the use of CONSORT guidelines whenever the results of randomised controlled trials are reported. The CONSORT guidelines were first published in 1996,[21] are now available on the web, and an updated version has recently been published.[22]

The CONSORT guidelines were established because of the growing recognition that randomised controlled trials are the best way to measure the effectiveness of treatments. These studies therefore need to be reported to an exceptionally high standard so that readers can judge whether the results are reliable.[23] The revised guidelines[22] are written in a clearer and more friendly language than before. They include a comprehensive checklist and a model flow chart diagram to help researchers publish the results of randomised controlled trials fully and accurately. The 22-item checklist which is summarised in Table 2.2 ensures that readers are well informed about the study methods, the results, and the analyses of the trial data, including the methods used for randomisation and allocation concealment.

The new guidelines have more precise requirements for explaining the flow of participants through a trial. Authors are asked to specify the number of participants in each of four phases of a trial, that is enrolment, intervention allocation, follow up, and analysis in a flow diagram. The flow diagram is designed to track patients through these stages to ensure that the number eligible for the trial, recruited, randomised to groups, and who completed the trial or were lost to follow up, is clear. These diagrams have an important function in improving the quality of the reporting of randomised controlled trials because they provide comprehensive counts of participants who pass through the various stages of recruitment.[24] Examples of flow diagrams can be seen in any of the major journals that publish randomised controlled trials. Figure 2.2 shows a typical flow chart from a randomised controlled trial.

Reports using the CONSORT guidelines will include all of the important study details, so that readers are readily able to judge whether any biases have influenced the study results.[26] Other guidelines are also available for assessing the quality of controlled clinical trials.[27] A statement has also been written for the reporting of meta-analyses of data from cross-sectional, case series, case–control, and cohort studies. This statement is called Meta-analysis of Observational Studies in Epidemiology (MOOSE) (www[7]). The MOOSE checklist outlines details of how background and search strategies as well as methods, results, discussions, and conclusions should be reported in meta-analyses of observational studies.[28] Use of this checklist will improve the value of meta-analyses to everyone who uses them.

Similarly, meta-analysts have developed the Quality of Reporting of Meta-analyses (QUOROM) statement.[29] The QUOROM statement has its own checklists and flow diagrams for reporting the methods used both to analyse the data from the journal articles reviewed and in the research articles

Table 2.2 CONSORT checklist of items to include when reporting a randomised controlled trial.[22]

Item	No.	Descriptor
Title and abstract	1	How participants were allocated to interventions (for example "random allocation", "randomised" or "randomly assigned")
Introduction		
Background	2	Scientific background and explanation of rationale
Methods		
Participants	3	Eligibility criteria for participants and the settings and locations where the data were collected
Interventions	4	Precise details of the interventions intended for each group and how and when they were actually administered
Objectives	5	Specific objectives and hypotheses
Outcomes	6	Clearly defined primary and secondary outcome measures and, when applicable, any methods used to enhance the quality of measurements (for example multiple observations, training of assessors, etc.)
Sample size	7	How sample size was determined and, when applicable, explanation of any interim analyses and stopping rules
Randomisation		
Sequence generation	8	Method used to generate the random allocation sequence, including details of any restriction (for example blocking, stratification)
Allocation concealment	9	Method used to implement allocation sequence (for example numbered containers or central telephone), clarifying whether the sequence was concealed until interventions were assigned
Implementation	10	Who generated the allocation sequence, who enrolled participants, and who assigned participants to their groups

(Continued)

Table 2.2 Continued.

Item	No.	Descriptor
Blinding (masking)	11	Whether or not participants, those administering the interventions, and those assessing the outcomes were aware of group assignment. If not, how the success of masking was assessed
Statistical methods	12	Statistical methods used to compare groups for primary outcome(s); methods for additional analyses, such as subgroup analyses and adjusted analyses
Results		
Participant flow	13	Flow of participants through each stage (a diagram is strongly recommended). Specifically, for each group, report the numbers of participants randomly assigned, receiving intended treatment, completing the study protocol, and analysed for the primary outcome. Describe protocol deviations from study as planned, together with reasons
Recruitment	14	Dates defining the period of recruitment and follow up
Baseline data	15	Baseline demographic and clinical characteristics of each group
Numbers analysed	16	Number of participants (denominator) included in each analysis and whether the analysis was by "intention to treat". State the results in absolute numbers when feasible (for example 10/20 not 50%)
Outcomes and estimation	17	For each primary and secondary outcome, a summary of results for each group, and the estimated effect size and its precision (for example 95% CI)
Ancillary analyses	18	Address multiplicity by reporting any other analyses performed, including subgroup analyses and adjusted analyses, indicating those prespecified and those exploratory
Adverse events	19	All important adverse events or side effects in each intervention group
Discussion		
Interpretation	20	Interpretation of the results, taking into account study hypotheses, sources of potential bias or imprecision, and the dangers associated with multiplicity of analyses and outcomes
Generalisability	21	Generalisability (external validity) of the trial findings
Overall evidence	22	General interpretation of the results in the context of current evidence

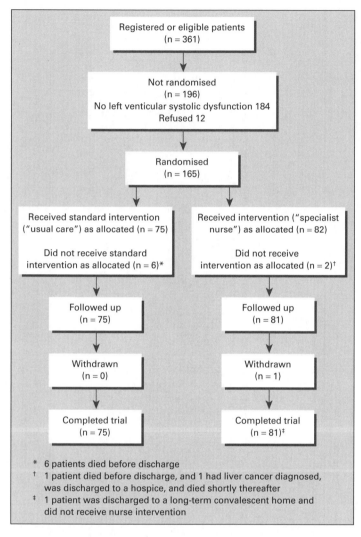

Figure 2.2 Typical flow chart of a randomised controlled trial of specialist nurse intervention in heart failure. Produced with permission from L Blue *et al. BMJ* 2001;**323**:715–18[25].

analysed (www[8]). The QUOROM statement includes recommendations for a structured abstract, and sections on validity assessment, data abstraction, study characteristics, and quantitative data synthesis.

Guidelines for authors and reviewers of qualitative studies have recently been published.[30] Further guidelines for reporting studies that are designed to assess diagnostic tests (STARD) and for reporting case–control and cohort studies are currently underway.[31] Details can be found at the *JAMA* website (www[9]).

The Cochrane Collaboration has developed a standard format for writing protocols and full versions of systematic reviews for publication in the Cochrane Library (www[10]). Specific software called Review Manager® is also available for standardising the analyses and representation of data (www[11]). Anyone interested in the Cochrane Collaboration should use the Cochrane website to contact their local Cochrane centre. It is important to note that publication of systematic reviews in the Cochrane Library does not exclude publishing the information as an article in a journal.

Authorship

> *It is a contradiction to be a co-author but then plead ignorance and assume victim status if there is controversy regarding data in the paper.*
>
> P de Sa, A Sagar[32]

Authorship is about publicly putting your name to your research achievements. Academics reap many personal and professional rewards from their research activity in general and their publications in particular. Authorship has a strong currency that brings not only personal satisfaction but also career rewards based on publication counting. Both the number of publications and the quality of the journal are often used to judge research reputations, to assess achievement for promotion, and to measure "track record" for granting bodies who allocate research funds. For these reasons alone, researchers rarely turn down an opportunity to coauthor a paper.

With so much at stake, making a decision about authorship can be the most sensitive part of writing a paper. In recognition of this, standard criteria for authorship have been developed. Whatever criteria are used, authorship should always be linked to an identifiable contribution. Journal editors often despair about authorship lists that include people who have done little, if anything, towards the conduct of the study and exclude people who have done much work, even if they cannot claim responsibility for the entire study.[33]

It is smart to make decisions about who will be authors and the order in which they will be placed before you begin writing or, even better, before the actual study gets underway. Early decisions tend to be less problematic than decisions made later, because the potential for conflict increases as the rewards attached to authorship increase and coworkers jockey for a higher position in the pecking order. At the Harvard Medical School, authorship disputes constituted 2·3% of issues presented to the ombudsman's office in 1991–92 and rose to 10·7% in 1996–97.[34] In trying to avoid such problems, early decisions about authorship can be an effective, preventive measure. An early decision can clarify the expectations of the research team and avoid the disappointment that inevitably occurs when people live in the hope of an authorship that never eventuates. It is certainly a mistake to put off authorship decisions in the hope that any ill feelings will eventually resolve of their own accord.

Authorship is best decided with the use of standard guidelines rather than reliance on an ad hoc grace and favour system. Many research teams use the widely renowned Vancouver guidelines[19] shown in Box 2.3. These guidelines were developed using the wide experience of several senior journal editors with the explicit aim of avoiding honorary and irresponsible authorship. Many journals and the Cochrane Collaboration ask authors to follow these guidelines.

Box 2.3 Vancouver guidelines on authorship[19]

Each author should have participated sufficiently in the work to take full responsibility for the content.
Authorship credit should be based only on:

a. substantial contributions to conception and design, or analysis and interpretation of data; and to
b. drafting the article or revising it critically for important intellectual content,
c. final approval of the version to be published.

Conditions a, b, and c must all be met. Any part of an article critical to its main conclusions must be the responsibility of at least one author. Editors may require authors to justify the assignment of authorship.

Despite wide recommendations for use of the guidelines, many research groups do not necessarily use them, often because they find them quite restrictive.[35] It has also been suggested that guidelines for authorship should not be externally imposed but should be developed in house by senior researchers in collaboration with their team.[36] Because the Vancouver guidelines require that authors conform to all three criteria rather than one or more of them, they may encourage researchers to exaggerate the contributions of colleagues, perhaps for their own career development.[37] It is widely agreed that participating solely in the acquisition of funding, the collection of data or the general supervision of the research team does not justify authorship. However, the Vancouver guidelines do not address the problem of researchers who have contributed to the work but whose names are not included as authors.[38]

Deciding where to draw authorship lines can be contentious in studies in which many people each make a specialised contribution, and large research teams often decide that meeting only one or two of the Vancouver criteria is sufficient. This more encompassing approach means that junior team members who are being trained into more senior roles need not be excluded. Also, by planning a series of publications from a single study, junior staff or students can be included as an author in at least one paper to which they are able to make an intellectual contribution. This provides an invaluable training opportunity and a way of sharing the rewards of authorship with the entire team. Some other ways in which data sharing can be handled in large research teams are discussed in Chapter 6.

A template for the order in which some of the political issues surrounding authorship, acknowledgements and choices of journal can be considered is shown in Figure 2.3.

The first author is always responsible for putting the paper together. As such, the first author makes decisions about the main aims of the paper in consultation with the coauthors. Until this is achieved, writing should not begin. The first author is also responsible for conducting or supervising the data analyses and ensuring that the results are presented and interpreted correctly. The supportive responsibilities of the coauthors are shown in Box 2.4. In effect, each author must be able to present the results, defend the implications,

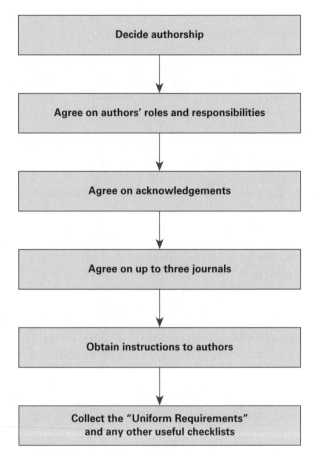

Figure 2.3 Sorting out the politics before you begin writing.

and discuss the limitations of the study to the professional research community and to the public, if need be. These responsibilities protect coauthors and preclude "gift" authors, since no researcher should allow their names to be associated with results that they know very little about.

Box 2.4 Responsibilities of authors and coauthors

First author

Takes primary responsibility for all aspects of publishing the paper
Conducts or supervises the data analyses and interprets the results
Writes the paper in consultation with coauthors
Maintains ownership of the master document
Submits the paper to a journal and deals with the correspondence
Responsible for archiving and documenting all data and files

Coauthors

Make early decisions about the aims of the paper
Keep the paper on track in terms of the main messages
Make intellectual contributions to the data analyses
Contribute to the interpretation of the results
Review each draft
Take public responsibility for the content and results

The list of coauthors may include team members, such as the statistician, database manager, librarian, study coordinator, and student supervisor. Box 2.5 shows the types of contributions that research team members may make to a paper. Whatever their positions in the author list, coauthors always have both ethical and professional responsibilities for the content of the paper. Thus, only the people who have participated sufficiently in the research project to take public responsibility for the content should be included. Once the authorship list is finalised, you can work towards an agreement on the role of each coauthor and the work that they will put into the paper. There are no formal guidelines so you will have to negotiate your expectations with those of your coauthors.

Box 2.5 Examples of intellectual contributions to a paper

Conception and design of the study
Implementation and data collection
Library searches and assembling relevant literature
Database management
Analysis and interpretation of the data
Writing and critical review of the paper
Supervising writing of a paper by a student

Table 2.3 Suggested maximum number of authors

Type of publication	Suggested maximum number of authors
Journal articles	8–9
Letters	4–5
Reviews	3–4

It is best to limit authorship to colleagues who make a true academic contribution. Although the number of authors on journal articles has tended to increase in recent years, four or five authors is usually optimal. Limiting the number of authors may be particularly important for the career advancement of students who are undertaking a higher degree and who are required to make a very substantial contribution to their papers. Having fewer authors also avoids diluting the responsibility that each author must take for the paper. In practice, more than four authors should be included only if there is a good reason for doing so and some journals set author limits. For example, the journal *Thrombosis and Haemostasis* sets a limit of eight and *Chest* sets a limit of seven. The *New England Journal of Medicine* sets a limit of 12 authors, after which other names must appear in a footnote. A suggested maximum number of authors for each type of publication is shown in Table 2.3.

A study on multiple authorship showed that the mean number of authors on journal articles increased from 2·2 in 1975 to 4·5 in 1995, with a disproportionate growth in the inclusion of professors and departmental chairpersons.[39] This supports the commonly held belief that homage in the form of automatic authorship should be paid to researchers who obtained funding for a study and to heads of departments.

Some journals, for example *JAMA* and the *New England Journal of Medicine*, now ask authors to certify that they meet the Vancouver criteria when a paper is submitted, and many journals include these criteria in their instructions to authors. Journals such as the *BMJ* and *Lancet* also request a statement of each author's exact contribution to the paper. To avoid authorship problems, research groups need to develop a departmental policy on authorship criteria that is regularly visited, discussed, and updated in a consensus forum. Many research institutions also develop their own code of ethics for acknowledgements and contributions in publications. Standardised policies that are developed collaboratively and ratified by the heads of research departments within institutions are worth their weight in gold in preventing conflicts and resolving contentious and often emotional authorship and acknowledgement issues.

Because authorship is such a serious issue, many journals will not consider a paper for publication without the signatures of all authors. Most journals also require a declaration of competing interests from their authors and contributors. The *Lancet* in its instructions to authors suggests that authors use the following statement:

> *I declare that I participated in the (here list contributions made to the study such as design, execution or analysis of the paper) by … and colleagues entitled … and that I have seen and approved the final version.*

It is also a good idea to add "I also declare that I have no conflict of interest in connection with this paper other than any noted in the covering letter to the editor". If these statements are completed on separate pages and left undated, they can be used if the paper is rejected and then submitted to another journal.

Authors must have independence and must be accountable. There have been cases where pharmaceutical companies have applied undue pressure on researchers to avoid publishing data that suggest that their products are inferior or ineffective. In response to what editors perceive as increasing control by drug companies over how the results of sponsored studies are analysed, many journals now require that authors fully disclose their own roles and those of their sponsors. Some major medical journals will not review or publish articles based on studies that are conducted under conditions that allow the sponsor to have sole control of the data or to withhold publication.[40] The journals that are members of the ICMJE now routinely require authors to disclose details of their own role and that of their sponsor.[41] Authors are asked to sign a statement that they accept full responsibility for the conduct of the study, had access to the data, and controlled the decision to publish. If the authors cannot satisfy these points, the paper will not be published. These moves are intended to prevent the publication of research results that reflect their financial backing.

Role of statisticians

> *A statistician is a person who likes to prove you wrong, 5% of the time.*
>
> Taken from an internet bulletin board

Statisticians often have a special place in the authorship of a paper that reflects their contribution to the design and/or reporting of the study. As such, they are a good example of how a person with specific expertise can support a study in either a minor or a major way. A statistician's role may vary from the development of the study design and study protocol to helping prepare the grant application, implementing the study, planning and performing the data analyses, and/or interpreting the results. Table 2.4 shows a scoring system that gives points for statistical contribution to various aspects of a study, and that can be used to decide whether a statistician's contribution warrants authorship.[42] Using this system, 5 points or fewer do not warrant authorship, 6–7 points indicate possible authorship and 8 or more points indicate certain authorship. In general, authorship is not warranted when the statistician has contributed to only one or two aspects of the paper in an entirely consultative way. However, authorship is often warranted when the statistician has been more actively involved and has made a fundamental, intellectual contribution that fulfils at least some of the Vancouver guidelines.

Author order

> *There is intense international competition in science these days which is a kind of substitute for war.*
>
> Gordon Lil and Arthur Maxwell (Science, 1959)

An additional problem in deciding authorship can be the order in which coauthors are listed. The first author is always

Table 2.4 Checklist for assessing statistical contribution to a study.[42]

Contribution	Points if involved
Study design	
Substantive input into the overall design of the study and protocol development ("thinking through a study")	4
Writing one or more sections of the grant applications (data analysis, data management)	2
Overall review of grant application prior to submission	1
Implementation	
Regular (ongoing) participation in study meetings with other investigators	4
Implementation of data collection and data management activities, including monitoring and supervision of data collection staff	2
Advising only on specific issues when requested by principal investigator ("answers only specific questions")	1
Analysis	
Planning and directing the analyses (usually based on analysis plan described in grant but includes exact model specification, resolution at decision points, etc.)	4
Preparing written material that summarises the results of the analysis for the other investigators and/or preparing formal reports	2
Doing the data analyses	1

the person who does the writing and who coordinates the team of coauthors. The last author is usually the senior member of the team and is often the person who conceived the initial idea for the study and/or obtained funding. It is common policy that the authors in between the first and last are ranked in order of the magnitude of their input into the paper.[43] However, there is no consensus on these widely used positions. On some papers, the last author may be the person who contributed the least in intellectual terms rather than the most. The Cochrane Collaboration specifically asks that the order reflects the size of the contribution made by each author so that the last author is the person who makes the smallest contribution.

In some cases, authorship lists are extremely long but are justified by the need for collaboration between centres as happens, for example, in international and multicentre studies. In recent years, new methods of acknowledging teams rather than individuals and of grouping contributors have been developed as shown in Box 2.6. However, teams should be aware that bibliographic databases vary in the way in which they list authors of multicentre studies. MEDLINE® often puts "no authors listed" and includes the name of the collective authorship in the title. At the other end of the scale, EMBASE® lists the names of up to 19 authors drawn from the byline before *et al.* is added, which sometimes results in authorship being attributed only to contributors with a surname at the beginning of the alphabet.[44] With the "cite six" Vancouver rule that recommends that only the first six authors are listed followed by an "*et al.*", many authors see particular merit in being high in the author list.

Box 2.6 Methods of acknowledging research teams in authorship lists

for the CAPS team[45]
for the ORACLE Collaborative Group[46]
for the European Community Respiratory Health Survey[47]
for the Evidence-Based Working Group[48]
for the Southampton NLU Evaluation Team[49]
and Contributors to the Australian Paediatric Surveillance Unit[50]

In an attempt to defuse the competition for authorship, various suggestions have been made for computing "publication equivalents" in a way that is fairer for assessing the track records of researchers. Some suggestions include dividing the author's rank in the authorship list by the sum of the ranks for all authors,[51] dividing each publication unit by the number of authors,[52] or attributing a proportion of the productivity to each author.[53,54] These systems, which effectively reduce a publication unit to a fraction that gets smaller as the number of authors increases, provide an incentive to minimise the number of coauthors. However, it is ironic that attempts to minimise author lists contradicts the current trend of universities, hospitals, and granting bodies to promote collaboration between research groups.

Some research groups write their own formal policies for deciding authorship. A policy entitled "The money, fame and happiness document" has been developed by a clinical research unit in Sydney and is given to all new researchers who join the unit (www[12]). This policy acknowledges the Vancouver guidelines for authorship but includes an algorithm for allocating points for specific contributions to a research project as shown in Box 2.7. The policy states that the Vancouver guidelines do not need to be used for most papers but that they are helpful at times when authorship decisions are difficult to make. The policy also gives advice on how to circumvent and resolve authorship problems and includes a statement that the organisation reserves the right to publish important reports without an author rather than waste the product of research conducted using public money. This policy may not suit all research units. What is important is that policies are developed in a collaborative way, are regularly revisited and revised if necessary, and are available to all potential authors.

Box 2.7 Credit point system for deciding authorship (www[12])

Algorithm for credit for work on a research project		Points
Initiation phase		
Ideas plus literature review plus hypotheses plus grant application		3
Pilot phase		
Development of instruments plus pilot plus reliability		2
Execution phase		
Management and key workers		1
Analysis phase		
Analysis design plus paper design plus draft write-up plus final write-up plus revisions		4
Points required for name on a paper		
Solo author		10
Two authors	1st	6
	2nd	4
Three authors	1st	5
	2nd	3
	3rd	2
Four authors	1st	5
	2nd	2, etc.

Without any internationally recognised standard criteria for author order, no system seems fair. Senior researchers are occasionally criticised for being only second or final authors when the system of using author order as an acknowledgement of mentoring, intellectual, and/or management credentials is not recognised. Until a consensus on the meaning of author order is achieved, researchers who strive to gain recognition for their own intellectual contribution whilst mentoring junior staff in the processes of writing and publication will always be disadvantaged. To deal with this issue, researchers applying for promotion often specify the exact contributions that they made to publications listed in their curriculum vitae.

Gift, ghost, and guest authors

Ghost writing is what you do for a football player when it is painfully obvious from his every utterance on and off the field that he has little to say but still needs help to say it.

David Sharp[55]

"Gift" authorship occurs when someone who has not made an intellectual contribution to a paper accepts an authorship. This type of authorship often develops because both the author and the "gift" author benefit from the relationship. Senior "gift" authors are often enrolled because they tend to confer a stamp of authority on a paper.[38] The "gift" author may gain prestige by being associated with the publication, and the author may gain approval for their work from the senior academic. Many researchers are willing to cite senior authors if they think that this will facilitate the publication of their work or enhance their career prospects.[56] However, this practice can lead to scandal when the results of a journal article cannot be substantiated.[57] For this reason, a head of department or a senior academic should not be included as an author when they have not made an academic contribution to the paper and are not able to take responsibility for the content. Most of all, gift authors should definitely not be included "because everyone does it".[38]

"Ghost" authorship, on the other hand, is the practice of omitting authors who have made a major contribution to a paper. In a survey of journal articles published in three peer-reviewed journals (*Annals of Internal Medicine, JAMA*, and the *New England Journal of Medicine*) in 1996, 11% of articles involved the use of ghost authors and 19% had evidence of honorary authors.[58] Professional ghost authors, or writers as most would call them, are sometimes engaged to write papers on which a clinical investigator, or "guest" author, is included but has not been involved in the data analyses or preparation of the manuscript.[59] This practice is most often attributed to drug companies who may pressure writers to use certain phrases to position a product more favourably.[60] Such practices may also be used to fast track the publication of clinical drug trials, but they reduce the independence of the research team and they do not conform in any way to the Vancouver guidelines. Although "guest" authors may have final control over the manuscript, they may not thoroughly review the paper if it does not have high priority in their workload. Given that science must be based on truth and trust, practices of "gift" and "ghost" authorship are to be avoided at all costs.

Contributions

> *If you haven't done the work, don't put your name on it.*
> *If you put your name on the paper, then you are stuck with it.*

CF Wooley[61]

The issues of whether, and how, contributors other than the authors of a paper should be listed and have their role acknowledged continues to be debated. This issue becomes especially problematic in the case of large multicentre trials. As a result, there has been a move towards some papers including guarantors and contributors instead of authors[62] and some journals now publish a byline disclosure of multicentre trials with a list of clinicians and study-organisation contributors, and a statement of the contribution of each author.

A move to naming "contributors" rather than authors was suggested to improve both the credibility and the accountability of authorship lists[62] and some large multicentre studies have adopted this approach. Journals such as the *Lancet* and the *BMJ* now list the contributions of researchers to some journal articles, often when the number of authors exceeds a prespecified threshold. However, in *JAMA* and in other journals, studies are often published with more than 40 authors who are listed in alphabetical order. Whereas some journal editors and readers see long lists of contributors as a way to reward and encourage researchers, others see it as wasted space.

As Box 2.8 shows, the tasks that constitute contribution to a Cochrane review are clearly defined. When the review is submitted, contributors are asked to describe in their own words their exact role in the review and this statement of contribution is then made available to readers. By defining the roles that constitute contribution rather than authorship, the Cochrane Collaboration have gone some way to helping solve authorship problems and ensuring that contributors are acknowledged appropriately.

Box 2.8 Examples of contributions to a Cochrane review (www[13])

Conceiving the review
Designing the review
Coordinating the review
Data collection for the review
   Developing the search strategy
   Undertaking searches
   Screening search results
   Organising retrieval of journal articles
   Screening retrieved journal articles against inclusion criteria
   Appraising quality of journal articles
   Abstracting data from journal articles
   Writing to authors of journal articles for additional information
   Providing additional data about journal articles
   Obtaining and screening data on unpublished studies
Data management for the review
   Entering data into RevMan
Analysis of data
Interpretation of data
   Providing a methodological perspective
   Providing a clinical perspective
   Providing a policy perspective
   Providing a consumer perspective
Writing the review
Providing general advice on the review
Securing funding for the review
Performing previous work that was the foundation of a current study

Acknowledgements

> *By all means recognise secretaries, wives or husbands,*
> *lovers and parents – but not in the manuscript.*

Alastair Spence[63]

Deciding who to formally acknowledge in your paper requires almost as much consideration as deciding authorship and contribution, although the criteria are less contentious. Some roles that commonly receive acknowledgement are shown in Box 2.9. Basically, all research and support staff who make a direct contribution to a study but who do not fulfil the criteria for authorship or contributorship should be granted a formal acknowledgement. Some journals require that people who are named in this section give permission to be acknowledged, preferably in writing, and that their specific contribution is described. If someone in the team has made a fundamental contribution to your study, it is naturally polite to acknowledge this contribution in a formal way.

Box 2.9 Contributions to a paper that warrant acknowledgement

General support by a department head or an institution
Technical help, laboratory work, and data collection
Input of students, trainees, and research assistants
Provision of clinical details of patients
Statistical, graphics, or library support
Critical review of the drafts
Financial support from granting bodies, drug companies etc.
Financial interests that may pose a conflict of interest

To decide whether to include your coworkers as authors, contributors, or acknowledgements, you can consult the Vancouver Group's criteria that are published under the ICMJE acronym.[19] or www[3] You can also consult your department policy, obtain the instructions to authors for your journal of choice, and look at previous examples of articles in the journal.

To limit the size of the acknowledgement list, the *New England Journal of Medicine* has developed a policy of publishing only a list that can fit into a single print column[64]; however, the acknowledgement pages in the *Lancet* are sometimes longer than one full page.

Acknowledgements

King quotes have been reprinted with the permission of Scribner, a Division of Simon & Schuster, Inc., from *On Writing: A Memoir of the Craft* by Stephen King. Copyright © by Stephen King. The Lil and Maxwell quote has been produced with permission from Horvitz, LA ed. *The Quotable Scientist.* New York: McGraw-Hill Companies, 2000 (p 5). All other referenced quotes have been produced with permission.

Websites

1 *BMJ* (*British Medical Journal*)
http://www.bmj.com/advice/index.html
Advice to authors and contributors on many issues on how to prepare papers for submission including checklists, copyright, defining ethnicity, writing advice, etc.

2 *Index Medicus*, United States National Library of Medicine
http://www.nlm.nih.gov/tsd/serials/lji.html
Bibliographic information including standard abbreviations for serials indexed and cited in MEDLINE®

3 International Committee of Medical Journal Editors (ICMJE)
http://www.icmje.org
Uniform requirements that provide instructions to authors on how to prepare manuscripts to submit to biomedical journals including links to sites about sponsorship, authorship, and accountability

4 Institute for Scientific Information
http://www.isiresearchsoft.com
Comparison of the features of the three most widely used bibliographic software programs EndNote®, Reference Manager®, and ProCite®

5 Medical College of Ohio, Raymon H. Mulford Library
http://www.mco.edu/lib/instr/libinsta.html
Links to websites that provide instructions to authors for over 2000 journals in the health sciences

6 Consolidated Standards of Reporting Trials
http://www.consort-statement.org/revisedstatement.htm
Guidelines for reporting randomised controlled trials (CONSORT)

7 Consolidated Standards of Reporting Trials
http://www.consort-statement.org/moose.pdf
Guidelines for reporting Meta–analysis of Observational Studies in Epidemiology (MOOSE)

8 Consolidated Standards of Reporting Trials
http://www.consort-statement.org/quorom.pdf
Guidelines for Quality of Reporting of Meta-analyses (QUOROM)

9 *JAMA (Journal of the American Medical Association)*
http://jama.ama-assn.org/issues/
Guidelines for writing papers reporting the results of diagnostic tests, cohort studies or case–control studies

10 Cochrane Collaboration
http://www.cochrane.org
Guidelines for authors and contributors for preparing systematic reviews of the effects of healthcare interventions

11 Cochrane Collaboration
http://www.cochrane.org/cochrane/revman.htm
Access to the Cochrane Collaboration's program RevMan for preparing and maintaining Cochrane reviews

12 University of New South Wales at St Vincent's Hospital, Clinical Research Unit for Anxiety and Depression
http://www.crufad.org
Access to "The money, fame and happiness document"

13 Cochrane Collaboration
http://www.update-software.com/ccweb/cochrane/hbook.htm
Access to the Cochrane Collaboration handbook

References

1 Rennie D, Flanagin A. Authorship! Authorship! Guests, ghosts, grafters, and the two sided coin. *JAMA* 1994;**271**:469–71.
2 Hall GM. Structure of a scientific paper. In: *How to write a paper*. London: BMJ Books, 1994; pp 1–5.
3 King S. *On writing*. London: Scribner, 2000; pp 114.
4 Fowkes FGR, Fulton PM. Critical appraisal of published research: introductory guidelines. *BMJ* 1991;**302**:1136–40.
5 Working group on recommendations for reporting clinical trials in the biomedical literature. Call for comments on a proposal to improve reporting of clinical trials in the biomedical literature. *Ann Intern Med* 1994;**121**:894–5.
6 Moyer VA. Confusing conclusions and the clinician: An approach to evaluating case-control studies. *J Pediatr* 1994;**124**:671–4.
7 Peat JK, Mellis CM, Williams K, Xuan W. Reviewing the literature. In: *Health science research. A handbook of quantitative methods*. London: Allen and Unwin, 2001; pp 1–12.
8 Fulginiti VA. On writing medical articles. *Am J Dis Child* 1983;**137**:620–1.
9 Editorial. Getting published in the BMJ: advice to authors. *BMJ* 1997;**314**:66–8.
10 Fontanarosa RB, Angelis CD. To JAMA peer reviewers and authors – thank you. *JAMA* 2003;**289**:756.
11 Williams ES. The *JAMA* peer review report for 2000. *JAMA* 2001;**285**:1078.
12 Macdonald G. The journal in 1996. *Aust NZ J Med* 1997;**27**:1.
13 Stern JM, Simes RJ. Publication bias: evidence of delayed publication in a cohort study of clinical research projects. *BMJ* 1997;**315**:640–5.

14 Bero LA, Glantz SA, Rennie D. Publication bias and public health policy on environmental tobacco smoke. *JAMA* 1994;**272**:133–6.

15 Duval S, Tweedie R. Practical estimates of the effect of publication bias in meta-analysis. *Australasian Epidemiologist* 1999;**5**:14–17.

16 Ioannidis JPA. Effect of the statistical significance of results on the time to completion and publication of randomized efficacy trials. *JAMA* 1998;**279**:281–6.

17 Misakian AL, Bero LA. Publication bias and research on passive smoking. *JAMA* 1998;**280**:250–3.

18 Frank E. Authors' criteria for selecting journals. *JAMA* 1994;**272**:163–4.

19 International committee of medical journal editors. Uniform requirements for manuscripts submitted to biomedical journals. *Ann Intern Med* 1997;**126**:36–47.

20 Smith R. Introductions. In: *How to write a paper.* Hall GM, ed. London: BMJ Books, 1994; p 8–13.

21 Begg C, Cho M, Eastwood S *et al.* Improving the quality of reporting of randomised controlled trials. The CONSORT statement. *JAMA* 1996;**276**:637–9.

22 Moher D, Schulz KF, Altman D, for the CONSORT group. The CONSORT statement: Revised recommendations for improving the quality of reports of parallel-group randomized trials. *JAMA* 2001;**285**:1987–91.

23 Altman DG. Better reporting of randomised controlled trials: the CONSORT statement. *BMJ* 1996;**313**:570–1.

24 Egger M, Juni P, Bartlett C, for the CONSORT group. Value of flow diagrams in reports of randomized controlled trials. *JAMA* 2001;**285**: 1996–9.

25 Blue L, Lang E, McMurray JJV *et al.* Randomised controlled trial of specialist nurse intervention in heart failure. *BMJ* 2001;**323**:715–18.

26 Levin A. Reporting standards and the transparency of trials. *Ann Intern Med* 2001;**134**:169–72.

27 Juni P, Altman DG, Egger M. Assessing the quality of controlled clinical trials. *BMJ* 2001;**323**:42–6.

28 Stroup DF, Berlin JA, Morton SC *et al.* Meta-analysis of observational studies in epidemiology. A proposal for reporting. *JAMA* 2000;**283**: 2008–12.

29 Moher D, Cook DJ, Eastwood S *et al.*, for the QUOROM Group. Improving the quality of reports of meta-analyses of randomised controlled trials: the QUOROM statement. *Lancet* 1999;**354**:1896–900.

30 Malterud K. Qualitative research: standard, challenges, and guidelines. *Lancet* 2001;**358**:483–8.

31 Rennie D. CONSORT revised – improving the reporting of randomized trials. *JAMA* 2001;**285**:2006–7.

32 de Sa P, Sagar A. "Struck" by fraud? *Science* 1996;**274**:1593.

33 Smith R. Open your eyes. *Lancet* 1998;**352**:898–9.

34 Wilcox LJ. The coin of the realm, the source of complaints. *JAMA* 1998;**280**:216–18.

35 Horton R, Smith R. Time to redefine authorship. *BMJ* 1996;**312**:723.

36 Van Der Weyden MB. Authorship: is there an identity crisis? *Med J Aust* 1997;**166**:623.

37 Bhopal R, Rankin J, McColl E *et al.* The vexed question of authorship: view of researchers in a British medical faculty. *BMJ* 1997;**314**:1009–10.

38 Smith J. Gift authorship: a poisoned chalice? *BMJ* 1994;**309**:1456–7.

39 Drenth JPH. Multiple authorship. The contribution of senior authors. *JAMA* 1998;**280**:219–21.

40 Davidoff F, DeAngelis CD, Drazen JM *et al.* Sponsorship, authorship and accountability. *JAMA* 2001;**286**:1232–3.

41 Smith R. Maintaining the integrity of the scientific record. *BMJ* 2001;**323**:588.
42 Parker RA, Berman NG. Criteria for authorship for statisticians in medical papers. *Stat Med* 1998;**17**:2289–99.
43 Savitz DA. What can we infer from author order in epidemiology? *Am J Epidemiol* 1999;**149**:401–3.
44 Chalmers I. The public interest. *Lancet* 1998;**352**:893–4.
45 Mihrshahi S, Peat JK, Webb K *et al.*, for the CAPS team. The Childhood Asthma Prevention Study (CAPS): Design and research protocol of a large randomised trial of the primary prevention of asthma. *Control Clin Trials* 2001;**22**:333–54.
46 Kenyon SL, Taylor DJ, Tarnow-Mordi W, for the ORACLE Collaborative Group. Broad-spectrum antibiotics for preterm, prelabour rupture of fetal membranes: the ORACLE I randomised trial. *Lancet* 2001;**357**:979–88.
47 Jarvis D, Chinn S, Lucsynska C, Burney P, for the European Community Respiratory Health Survey. The association between respiratory symptoms and lung function with the use of gas for cooking. *Eur Respir J* 1998;**11**:651–8.
48 Naylor CD, Guyatt GH, for the Evidence-Based Medicine Working Group. Users' guides to the medical literature. *JAMA* 1996;**275**:554–8.
49 Steiner A, Walsh B, Pickering RM, Wiles R, Ward J, Brooking JI, for the Southampton NLU Evaluation Team. Therapeutic nursing or unblocking beds? A randomised controlled trial of post acute intermediate care unit. *BMJ* 2001;**322**:453–60.
50 Elliott EJ, Robins-Browne RM, O'Loughlin EV *et al.* and contributors to the Australian Paediatric Surveillance Unit. Nationwide study of haemolytic uraemic syndrome: clinical, microbial and epidemiological features. *Arch Dis Child* 2001;**85**:125–31.
51 Rothman KJ. A proposal to calculate publication equivalents. *Epidemiology* 1999;**10**:664–5.
52 Marusic A, Marusic M. Authorship criteria and academic reward. *Lancet* 1999;**353**:1713–14.
53 Kapoor VK. Polyauthoritis giftosa. *Lancet* 1994;**346**:1039.
54 Digiusto E. Equity in authorship: a strategy for assigning credit when publishing. *Soc Sci Med* 1995;**38**:55–8.
55 Sharp D. A ghostly crew. *Lancet* 1998;**351**:1076.
56 Eastwood D, Derish P, Leash E, Ordway S. Ethical issues in biomedical research: perceptions and practices of postdoctoral fellows responding to a survey. *Sci Eng Ethics* 1996;**2**:89–114.
57 Court C. Obstetrician suspended after research inquiry. *BMJ* 1994;**309**:1459.
58 Flanagin A, Carey LA, Fontanarosa PB, Phillips SG, Lundberg GD, Rennie D. Prevalence of articles with honorary authors and ghost authors in peer-reviewed medical journals. *JAMA* 1998;**280**:222–4.
59 Bodenheimer T. Uneasy alliance. Clinical investigators and the pharmaceutical industry. *N Engl J Med* 2000;**342**:1539–44.
60 Larkin M. Whose article is it anyway? *Lancet* 1999;**354**:136.
61 Wooley CF. "Struck" by fraud? Science 1996;**274**:1593.
62 Rennie D, Yank V, Emanuel L. When authorship fails. A proposal to make contributors accountable. *JAMA* 1997;**278**:579–85.
63 Spence AA. Discussions. In: *How to write a paper*. Hall GM, ed. London: BMJ Books, 1994; pp 30–32.
64 Topol EJ. Drafter and draftees. *Lancet* 1998;**352**:897–8.

3: Writing your paper

> *Now, practically even better news than that of short assignments is the idea of shitty first drafts. All good writers write them. This is how they end up with good second drafts and terrific third drafts. People tend to look at successful writers ... and think that they sit down at their desks every morning feeling like a million dollars, feeling great about who they are and how much talent they have ... and that they take in a few deep breaths, push back their sleeves, roll their necks a few times to get all the cricks out, and dive in, typing fully formed pages as fast as a court reporter. But this is just the fantasy of the uninitiated. I know some very great writers, writers you love who write beautifully ... and not one of them sits down routinely feeling wildly enthusiastic and confident. None of them writes elegant first drafts.*
>
> Anne Lamott[1]

The objectives of this chapter are to understand how to:

- order your material
- construct a neat abstract
- write an effective introduction
- describe your methods so that other researchers could repeat your study
- report your results precisely
- make your discussion relevant and interesting

When you are writing a journal article, it is logical to begin by writing the methods and then the results sections. The introduction and discussion can be pieced together as you progress, and finally you will need to condense it all into an abstract. In this chapter, we explain how to write each part of a paper and we have presented the sections in the order in which they will ultimately appear in your paper, which is not necessarily the order in which they should be written.

Abstract

The shortest way to do many things is to only do one thing at once.

Samuel Smiles (1812–1904)

You must pay particular attention to writing the abstract of your paper. Your abstract is essential for providing a condensed, potted history of your results in a fraction of the words that you use in the paper. Like a Readers Digest Condensed Book, this section of your paper should only convey the most interesting and most important parts of your work. Ideally, your abstract will be added to a public database such as MEDLINE® or PubMed® and will therefore achieve a much wider distribution than the journal article itself. People don't read the whole article unless they have a vested interest in the topic and many people rely on reading the abstract to decide whether to obtain the entire article.

The abstract should be organised by first stating the aims of the study followed by the basic study design and methods. This should then be followed by the main results including specific data and their statistical significance. Finally, finish with the conclusion and interpretation.

To ensure that the abstract contains all of the necessary information, many journals now require that you structure your abstract formally. The *BMJ* suggests objectives, design, setting, participants, main outcome measures, results, and conclusions as the subheadings of its structured abstracts. Other journals, particularly journals that publish both clinical and laboratory studies, limit their abstract headings to the standard aims, methods, results, and conclusions. Even if the journal does not specify any subheadings, write your abstract as though they were there.

Box 3.1 shows an example of a concise and well-structured abstract. In this abstract, there are no wasted words or redundant phrases. The results are supported by data and P values. Finally, the interpretation of the findings is clearly stated in the conclusion.

> **Box 3.1 Example of a well-structured abstract**
>
> **Randomised controlled trial of specialist nurse intervention in heart failure[2]**
>
> **Objectives** To determine whether specialist nurse intervention improves outcome in patients with chronic heart failure.
> **Design** Randomised controlled trial.
> **Setting** Acute medical admissions unit in a teaching hospital.
> **Participants** 165 patients admitted with heart failure due to left ventricular systolic dysfunction. The intervention started before discharge and continued thereafter with home visits for up to 1 year.
> **Main outcome measures** Time to first event analysis of death from all causes or readmission to hospital with worsening heart failure.
> **Results** 31 patients (37%) in the intervention group died or were readmitted with heart failure compared with 45 (53%) in the usual care group (hazard ratio – 0·61, 95% confidence interval 0·33 to 0·96). Compared with usual care, patients in the intervention group had fewer readmissions for any reason (86 versus 114, $P = 0·018$), fewer admissions for heart failure (19 v 45, $P < 0·001$) and spent fewer days in hospital for heart failure (mean 3·43 v 7·46 days, $P = 0·0051$).
> **Conclusions** Specially trained nurses can improve the outcome of patients admitted to hospital with heart failure.

When writing your abstract, put your most concise and important sentences on a page, join them into an abstract and then count the words. Abstracts always benefit from a serious word trim. It is essential that you adhere to the word limit. Some journals such as *Science* and *Nature* that are very well regarded in scientific circles request very short abstracts, which may be as low as 100 words. However, the usual limit is 250 words. Even if a larger word count is allowed, limit yourself to 250 words. MEDLINE® accepts only 250 words before it truncates the end of the abstract and cuts off your most important sentences, that is the conclusion and interpretation in the final sentences. It is always amazing how many words you can leave out if need be. If you can't word trim yourself, ask a colleague to do it for you. Other people can often be more objective and ruthless than you can be with your own writing.

Introduction

> *Almost all good writing begins with terrible first efforts.*
> *You need to start somewhere. Start by getting something –*
> *anything – down on paper. A friend of mine says that the*
> *first draft is the down draft – you just get it down. The*
> *second draft is the up draft – you fix it up.*
>
> Anne Lamott[1]

Introductions should be short and arresting and tell the reader why you undertook the study.[3] The best introductions fit on one page. In essence, this section should be brief rather than expansive and the structure should funnel down from a broad perspective to a specific aim as shown in Figure 3.1.[4]

The first paragraph should be a very short summary of the current knowledge of your research area. This should lead directly into the second paragraph that summarises what other people have done in this field, what limitations have been encountered with work to date, and what questions still need to be answered. This, in turn, will lead to the last paragraph, which should clearly state what you did and why. This sequence is logical and naturally provides a good format in which to introduce your story.

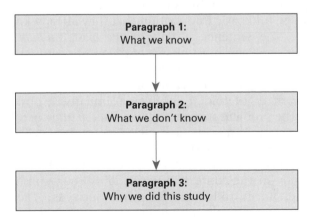

Figure 3.1 Template for the Introduction.

The introduction can be one of the hardest parts of a paper to write, but adopting this approach helps you to focus on how you want to start and what you specifically need to say. Most readers want a quick and snappy introduction to your work. Topic sentences, especially for the first introductory sentence, are a great help. These sentences are discussed in more detail in Chapter 8. Richard Smith, editor of the *BMJ*, stresses the importance of trying as hard as you can to hook your readers in the first line.[3] The introduction is where readers like to find the information that tells them exactly why you did the study. Few readers want to plough through a detailed history of your research area that goes over two or more pages.

In the introduction section, you do not need to review all of the literature available, although you do need to find it all and read it in the context of writing the entire paper. In appraising the literature, it is important to discard the scientifically weak studies and only draw evidence from the most rigorous, most relevant, and most valid studies. Ideally, you should have done a thorough literature search before you began the study and have updated it along the way. This will be invaluable in helping you to write a pertinent introduction.

You should avoid including a lot of material in the introduction section that would be better addressed in the discussion. You should never be tempted to put "text book" knowledge into your introduction because readers will not want to be told basic information that they already know. For example, the sentence, *Asthma is the most common chronic disease of childhood,* must be one of the most overused phrases in the last decade. All scientists working in asthma research and most people in the community already know this and don't want to be told it yet again. Similarly, a phrase that defines the problem such as, *Asthma is a condition in which the airways narrow in response to commonly occurring environmental stimuli,* is not appropriate, except in a paper about the mechanisms of airway narrowing. It is much better to put your study in the context in which it will be published. For example, an introductory sentence such as, *The mould Alternaria occurs ubiquitously in dry regions and is thought to be important in exacerbating symptoms of asthma,* defines the background behind this particular research study. In this sentence, the focus of the study and the cause of the exacerbations (Alternaria) rather than the disease itself (asthma) is the topic of the sentence, as it should be.

Do not be tempted to begin your introduction by quoting the literature but omitting to say what was found. For example, an introduction that begins with, *Previous studies have reviewed injury rates in Australian Army and RAAF recruits undergoing basic training. A study by Johnson* et al., *reviewed the medical records of Navy recruits who were unable to complete basic training* suggests that previous work has been undertaken in your research area. However, the lack of information about what was actually found does not help readers to put your work in the context of what has gone before. It is always better to quote the findings from previous studies rather than the name of the first author and the details of the aims or methods. For example, you could write, *Injury rates in Australian Army and RAAF recruits undergoing basic training were 12% per year in 1997 but were much higher at 47% in Navy recruits who were unable to complete basic training.* This sentence explains the prevalence of injuries at a specific point in time and, as such, quotes the science and not the scientist.

Before you can begin writing, you need to have an aim or a research question that is both novel and worth answering. The most essential part of the introduction is the last paragraph, which gives details of your aim or hypothesis. This is where the sentence that will dictate the content of the remainder of your paper should be found. This sentence sets up the expectations for the rest of the paper and should be the very first sentence that you write in collaboration with your coauthors. This is also a good place to tell your readers, in a few words, the type of study design that you used to test your hypothesis.

Finally, you should never end the introduction section with a quick summary of your own results. For example do not write, *We have undertaken a study to define the characteristics of children who become overweight. The results show that lack of exercise is a key factor and provide evidence that there has been a significant increase in overweight boys and girls in the last 12 years.* The practice of putting the key results at the end of the introduction section is common in some disciplines such as basic research but should not be used in clinical research. This type of misplaced summary stops the flow of the paper, makes it look disorganised and only serves to confuse the reader who has not yet been given enough information to make a judgement about the validity and applicability of the results.

Box 3.2 shows an example of an introduction that is short, to the point and gives a clear message about what we know (paragraph 1), what we don't know (paragraph 2) and the study methods that were therefore used (paragraph 3). This introduction is a little shorter than many in the literature in that it uses less than 160 words to get the important messages across. However, this brief introduction is to the point, and extra padding is not required.

Box 3.2 Example of an Introduction, which gives only essential information

Introduction

People who are overweight or obese are at increased risk of developing many illnesses including hypertension, cardiovascular disease, and non-insulin dependent diabetes. However, many adults continue to be overweight. In 1995, results from the National Nutrition Survey in Australia suggested that 63% of men and 47% of women were either overweight or obese.

Despite the impact of excess body weight on health, self-perception of body mass in the general population has not been properly investigated. The only information comes from small, unrepresentative samples of women, particularly younger women, or from national studies in which self-reported weights may be unreliable. Until reliable information of self-perceptions of body mass is collected, it is difficult to design effective weight loss intervention strategies.

In 1998, we conducted a large cross-sectional survey of adults in which we accurately measured height and weight. In this paper, we report information about adults' perceptions of their own body mass.

Methods

A rocket is an experiment; a star is an observation.

José Bergamín (1895–1983, www. bartelby.com)

The purpose of the methods section is to describe how you obtained your results. Thus, you need to give precise details of the study design, the methods that you used, and how you analysed the data. You should also give some information of where the study was conducted. When writing an epidemiological paper or a paper concerned with environmental issues, you may need to give some information about the locations of the centres where the data were collected. Be fairly circumspect in this. Remember that you are not writing a travel guide.

Every measurement reported in the results section must have a description of the method used to obtain it. This does not give you licence to fill many pages with all of the minute details of your study. The methods section should only be as long as is needed to describe the essential details. In reading this section, other researchers should be able to appraise your work critically or repeat your study exactly the way that you did it. The headings that are used in methods sections, such as participants, study design, specific methods, data analysis, etc. classically dictate their own content.

Ethical approval

> *Ethicists must exercise a constructive and objective gate-keeping function.*
>
> J Benson[5]

It is important to give the details of the institutional ethics review boards who approved your study. Readers will want to be assured that the welfare and rights of the participants in your study were placed above those of the investigators. Ethics committees are convened to protect the rights and welfare of research participants, to determine whether the risks to participants are warranted by the potential outcomes, and to ensure that informed consent is obtained. Because ethical approval is fundamental to good research practice, many journals now decline to publish results from studies that do not include details of prior ethical approval.

In a recent review of published articles, 40% of studies did not report ethical approval even though all five of the journals surveyed ask authors to document this.[6] As a result, recommendations were made to prevent unethical research being published in the future. The authors recommended that every research study should include a statement regarding human subjects and should not refer to other publications for information regarding ethical approval. If the investigators believed that their study did not need to be reviewed by an ethics committee, the reason for this exemption, which should not have been made by the authors themselves, should be provided. Investigators should always document both the approval from the ethics committee and whether informed consent was obtained from each participant. Because the protection of participants is one of the highest priorities in clinical research, every paper must contain a statement about the protection of the participants.[6]

Study design

> *Dream research is a wonderful field. All you do is sleep for a living.*
>
> Ann Fadiman (www.bartelby.com)

The study design should have been clearly identified before the study even began and should be easily described in the methods section. Table 3.1 shows the types of study design that are commonly used in health research.[7] It is important to state the design of your study up front because each study type has its own strengths and limitations in terms of controlling for bias or confounding. Each study design also dictates the type of statistical tests that are appropriate for analysing the data and describing the results. It may also be important to state whether your study was observational or experimental.

Participants

> *Research is a formalised curiosity. It is poking and prying with a reason.*
>
> Zora Neal Hurston (African-American novelist, 1891–1960, www.bartelby.com)

Table 3.1 Features of clinical and epidemiological quantitative research studies.

Study type	Characteristics	Method/s
Systematic or Cochrane review	• Review of the literature to answer a specific question about a therapy, intervention or exposure • Requires systematic, explicit search criteria to identify all published studies • Results from several studies may be combined statistically using a meta-analysis	Literature review Retrospective
Randomised controlled trial (RCT)	• Used to compare the effect of a new treatment with an existing or placebo treatment • Participants are allocated to study groups using a formal randomisation process • Randomisation minimises the effects of bias and confounding on the results	Experimental Prospective
Quasi- or non-randomised clinical trial	• Similar to an RCT but quasi- or non-random methods are used to allocate participants to groups • Quasi-randomisation methods include use of birth date, medical record number, etc. • Uncontrolled bias and confounding may influence the results	Experimental Prospective
Cohort study	• Data are collected from participants regularly over a long period of time • The development of disease in participants with different exposures is compared • Prognosis and/or causation can be inferred when an exposure is measured before an outcome • Most cohort studies are prospective, that is the cohort is enrolled and followed into the future	Observational Prospective or retrospective

(Continued)

Table 3.1 Continued

Study type	Characteristics	Method/s
Case–control study	• Cases with a disease of interest and controls who do not have the disease are enrolled • Differences in exposures or treatments between the cases and controls can be compared • Provides a fast, inexpensive way to measure risk factors • Bias and confounding are difficult to control and causation cannot be inferred	Observational
Cross-sectional studies	• A large, random selection of a defined population is enrolled • Participants have their health status, exposures etc., measured at a single point in time • Can be used to measure risk factors but causation cannot be inferred • Also called population or prevalence studies	Observational
Methodology studies	• Used to measure whether a test is accurate or can be used interchangeably with another test • Important for assessing the validity of research methods	Observational
Ecological studies	• Used to compare summary data such as prevalence rates, pollen counts etc., between populations • Bias and confounding cannot be controlled • Hypothesis generating only	Observational
Case reports	• Used to describe or summarise the records of interesting medical cases • Provide new information for clinicians and/or hypothesis generating	Observational

Readers will want to know how you recruited people into your study. In this, the sampling frame should be clearly described and the inclusion and exclusion criteria should be spelt out in detail. In describing the participants in your study, their privacy must always be respected. Do not include any identifying information in the text, tables, or photographs. Even masking the eyes in a photograph is insufficient to ensure anonymity. If a photograph is used, written consent must be obtained from the patient or their parent or guardian.

In describing the participants and the non-participants in your study, you should use accurate and sensitive descriptions of race and ethnicity and describe the logic behind any groupings that you use.[8] Common descriptors that can be used are gender, self-assigned ethnicity, observer-assigned ethnicity, country of birth, country of birth of parents, years in country of residence, and religion. If you want to describe the generalisability of your study, it is a good idea to use exactly the same descriptors that are used for the national census so that direct comparisons can be made. Such descriptors are often pragmatic in order to balance ease of collection against a need to collect data from an entire population.[9] This may result in having to use a multitude of descriptive terms but there is no simple way to classify all the people in a community into a narrow range of definitions.

Some researchers also include the sample size and sample characteristics in this part of the methods section although this information is probably better placed at the beginning of the Results section where most readers expect to find it.

Sample size

> *It is most important to have a beautiful theory. And if the observations don't support it, don't be too distressed, but wait a bit and see if some error in the observations doesn't show up.*

> Paul Dirac (theoretical physicist, 1980)

The size of your study sample is of paramount importance for testing your hypothesis or fulfilling the study aims. The number of participants in any study should be large enough to provide precise estimates of effect and therefore a reliable answer to the research question being addressed. You may be under some pressure to publish your work quickly, but your study should not be stopped or written up before an adequate number of participants has been recruited and studied. Even if formal sample size calculations suggested that you only needed a small number of participants, it is usually difficult to interpret the results from studies with fewer than 30 participants in each group. When the sample size is smaller than this, the results are rarely believable, the summary estimates lack precision, standard statistical methods may be inappropriate, and the generalisability of the results will be questionable. Providing a reliable answer to a study question usually means recruiting larger numbers of participants and, in terms of scientific integrity, it is worth going the hard yard to do this.

It is always important to include details of your sample size calculations. Your readers will need to know what outcome variables your study was designed to detect a difference in, what size of difference you initially expected, what power level you were working with, and why you chose a particular sample size. In practice, many studies with negative results do not have a large enough sample size to show that clinically important differences are statistically significant.[10] If this is the case, your readers will need this information in order to interpret your results appropriately. If your statistics lead you to accept the null hypothesis, having set up an experiment to disprove it, fellow scientists are entitled to information about the effect size that you considered clinically important at the outset. The probability that your findings were a result of type I and type II errors, which are explained in Box 3.3, needs to be made clear.

Box 3.3 Statistical terms used in sample size calculations

Type I errors

Errors that occur when a difference between groups is small and is not clinically important but reaches statistical significance. This usually happens because the study is overpowered in terms of sample size and the result is that the null hypothesis is rejected in error.

Type II errors

Errors that occur when a clinically important difference between two groups fails to reach statistical significance. This usually happens when the study is underpowered in terms of sample size and the result is that the null hypothesis is accepted in error.

Power

Chance of finding a statistically significant difference when there is one, or of rejecting the null hypothesis. A study with a power of 80% has a 20% chance of a type II error occurring.

Probability

Level at which a difference between groups is considered statistically significant, for example $P < 0.05$.

Questionnaires

> *Can you measure it? Can you express it in figures? Can you make a model of it? If not, your theory is apt to be based more upon imagination than upon knowledge.*

> William Thompson (physicist, 1927)

Many research studies use questionnaires to collect information about the participants' characteristics, exposure to environmental risk factors, current and previous illness history, and so on. In the methods section, you should give precise details of the questionnaires you used and how they were developed, validated, and tested for repeatability. The mode of administration must also be spelt out since different types of bias can arise when questionnaires are self-administered, telephone-administered, or interviewer-administered. A questionnaire that is thoughtfully designed has good face, content and construct, or criterion validity that minimises both measurement bias and the amount of missing or unusable information. If your questionnaire has been validated, always give a reference to the work.

Interventions

> *Science is facts. Just as houses are made of stones, so is science made of facts. But a pile of stones is not a house and a collection of facts is not necessarily science.*

> Jules Poincare (French scientist, 1854–1912,
> www.bartelby.com)

In experimental studies, details of the interventions and how they were administered need to be fully described. It is important to include exact details of the intervention of interest, and the intervention, sham, or placebo that was used for comparison. You must also describe the methods of randomisation, allocation concealment and blinding of the research staff and the participants to study group allocation. You must also describe any procedures that you used to maximise or measure compliance with the interventions. If a drug is being tested, then the generic name, the manufacturer, the doses used and any other information should be included.

Clinical assessments

Research is never completed ... Around the corner lurks another possibility of interview, another book to read, ... a document to verify.

Catherine Bowen (US biographer, 1897–1973, www.bartelby.com)

In this section, you must explain in detail the methods that you used to collect clinical information from the participants so that the study could be repeated if necessary. Most equipment that can be bought off the shelf is well known and can be described with a simple brand name and supplier. However, rare or newly devised equipment will need to be described in more detail. Only ever give a reference to a previous journal article to describe a method if the journal is freely available and if the article describes the method in a comprehensive way. It is sometimes a good idea to say why a particular method or piece of equipment was used and what advantages it had over other similar or more commonly used methods.

It is also important to include details of how equipment was calibrated and standardised if more than one piece of equipment was used. A critical issue in reducing bias in any study is the degree of comparability between items of equipment, between observers and within participants. This always needs to be addressed and explained.

Statistical methods

> *Like dreams, statistics are a form of wish fulfilment.*

> Jean Baudrillard (French seminologist, b. 1929,
> www.bartelby.com)

The statistical methods section should describe how you analysed the data with specific details of the statistical tests and the statistical computer packages that were used. Always give the P value that you used as the critical value to determine statistical significance. This is usually $P < 0.05$, although values such as $P < 0.01$ are common if multiple statistical tests are being conducted, and a critical level of $P < 0.1$ is sometimes used in multivariate modelling. Misunderstanding can occur if the critical P value is not stated.

Results can vary if the outcome or exposure variables are analysed as continuous, non-parametric, or categorical data. It is essential that you give as much information as possible about the distribution of your variables and the tests you use because serious bias can arise if the incorrect statistical test is used. In essence, readers need to know exactly how you obtained your results and why you came to the conclusions that you reached. If you used a statistical test that is not simple or well known, a reference to the method and an explanation of why you used it is required.

Results

> *Think of yourself as a reader for a moment. What kind of papers do you like to read? Short, meaty, and clear most likely. Well, then, write short, meaty, and clear papers yourself. Short, meaty and clear papers are most likely to be understood. The truth of this proposition will come home to you as you read biomedical writing and discover how easy it is to get the wrong message.*

> Mimi Zeiger[4]

This section is the most important part of your paper because its function is to give specific answers to the aims that you stated in the introduction. After the methods, this should be the easiest section to write. You should use an interesting sequence of text, tables, and figures to answer the study questions and to tell the story without diversions.

It is essential to know your audience and make it clear to them in their own language how your work is an important extension of what has gone before. In practice, editors usually prefer to publish new findings. Although consistency of evidence is critical for ascertaining causation,[11] most editors are not keen to publish results that are already thought of as established knowledge. It is important to convince the journal editor, your reviewers, and your readers that your study extends knowledge rather than merely confirms what we already know.

Figure 3.2 shows a template for the structure. The best way to present results is to gradually build up from univariate statistics to describe the characteristics of your study sample, through bivariate analyses to describe relationships between your explanatory and outcome variables, and finally to any multivariate analyses. This section should be quite straightforward and should guide your reader through your own discovery processes. The length of the section should be dictated entirely by how many results you have to present and not by how much you want to say about them.

Paragraph 1 of the results section should give accurate details of your study sample so that the generalisability of your results is clear. In most papers, Table 1 is used to describe the details of the participants. This is important because epidemiologists will want to know the defining characteristics of your sample and physicians will want to know if the participants in a clinical study are similar to their own patients.

Following paragraph 1, the next paragraphs will explain what your paper is really about because this is where you address the aims or test the hypothesis outlined at the end of the Introduction section. In writing these paragraphs, only tell the readers what they need to know. Do not be tempted to add asides or include any data analyses that are drifting away from the main purpose. Topic sentences that begin each paragraph are useful for this. Table 3.2 shows an example of how to use topic sentences to guide the reader through a results section.

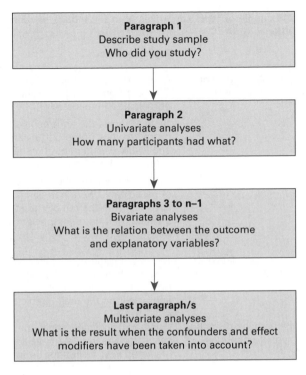

Figure 3.2 Template for the Results.

Remember that results and data are not the same thing. You do not need to repeat numbers in the text that are already presented in a table or a figure. A good trick to improve readability is to describe what you found in the text and then back it up with results that are shown in a figure or a table. For example, to describe the data shown in Figure 3.3 you can say that, *The figure shows that significantly more children with persistent cough had ever used an asthma medication or had used a bronchodilator or preventive medication in the last 12 months compared to asymptomatic children. However, medication use in children with persistent cough was significantly lower than in children with wheeze (P < 0·001).* The figure shows the prevalence of medication use in each group so that exact percentages do not need to be included in the text.

Table 3.2 Example of topic sentences from the results section of a cross-sectional study.[12]

Notes	Topic sentences
The first paragraphs describe who the participants were.	A total of 1527 participants aged 18 to 73 years from two rural regions participated in this study.
	Table 1 shows the anthropometric characteristics of the participants ... and Figure 1 illustrates the selection criteria for our normal group.
	Table 2 shows that the "normal" group of participants were not significantly different from the remainder of the sample in terms of age, height, and weight ($P > 0.05$).
The next paragraph describes the bivariate analyses.	The data for the normal group were used to obtain regression equations for FVC, FEV_1 ... with weight, age, gender, and height as the main predictors.
The next paragraphs describe how the bivariate analyses were used.	Using our prediction equations, we calculated mean percentage of predicted FEV_1 values for the whole sample (Figure 2).
	We then examined the factors that affect lung function.
The final paragraph describes the multivariate analyses.	Multiple regression showed that airway inflammation and asthma were significantly related to reductions in FEV_1 and that the interaction between airway inflammation and recent symptoms was also significant ($P < 0.05$).

Readers need to be given the messages that can be derived from a table or figure and should not be left to interpret the data themselves. If you want to compare your results with results from other studies, this comparison is better placed in the discussion section.

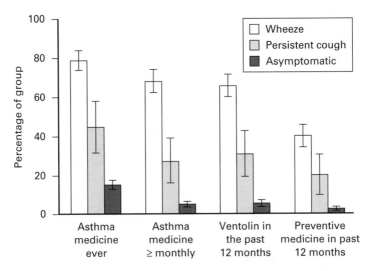

Figure 3.3 Persistent cough: is it asthma? Produced with permission from AO Faniran *et al. Arch Dis Child* 1998;**79**:411–14.[13]

Data analysis

> *Up to 2300 cars an hour use each lane of the M4 while figures show that Victoria Rd is flooded with more than 93,000 vehicles a day.*

> Daily Telegraph (18 April 2001)

It is essential that you are always consistent in the use of units in your reporting so that readers can make valid comparisons between and within groups. The media quote above, which uses different units of time and lane use for the two roadways, does not help us to decide which roadway is carrying the most traffic. You must avoid this type of problem in a scientific paper by carefully adhering to the correct measurements for the publication of research results. Most journals require you to use Système Internationale (SI) units although some American journals have different policies. For example, *JAMA* prefers imperial units of measurement with SI units being secondarily expressed in parentheses. Thus, plasma glucose concentrations are published in units of mg/dL instead of mmol/L and serum insulin concentrations are published in units of μIU/ml instead of pmol/L. As an author, you need to take great care when converting data from SI to conventional units or vice versa.

Data analysis is not always a straightforward process. Before you began your analyses, you should have classified your variables into the separate groups of outcome variables, intervening variables, and explanatory variables.[14] This will direct your data analyses along a sensible track.

Science is essentially an investigative process and, while you are trying to answer one research question, other questions or ideas often come to mind. When undertaking your data analyses, you may find answers to questions that you didn't expect, or you may find questions that you were not expecting to answer.[15] How you approach these extra analyses is a matter of ethics and pragmatics. Most researchers are happy if you conduct analyses that answer a question grounded in biological plausibility and for which the study design was entirely appropriate to answer the question. The use of an existing data set to explore ideas that emerge during the data analyses helps to conserve resources and maximise efficiency. However, it is wise to avoid producing spurious results or generating random significant findings by "data dredging" or by looking for associations between variables that are unlikely to be linked on causal pathways. It is a delicate balance, so proceed with care.

Baseline characteristics

Fate and character are the same thing.

Novalis (1772–1801)

To describe the baseline characteristics of the participants in any type of study, always use a table and never use a figure. In many experimental and observational studies, you will need to demonstrate the comparability of the study groups at baseline. The baseline characteristics also define the generalisability of your results. Thus, you need to describe the important characteristics of the study groups and show whether any potential confounders were unevenly distributed and were likely to cause an important bias that may have helped to explain the results. Never be tempted to call the baseline characteristics the "demographics" of your study sample. According to the *Shorter Oxford Dictionary*, demography is the branch of anthropology in which the statistics of births, deaths, and diseases are studied and is therefore not appropriate in this context.[15]

In randomised controlled trials, it is better to report descriptive statistics that show the distribution of the variable in each group, as shown in Table 3.3, rather than using formal statistical tests to determine if the differences between the groups were greater than would have been expected by chance. In any study, a percentage, the mean and its standard deviation, or the median and its interquartile range are the most appropriate descriptive statistics depending on the information that you are describing. In Table 3.3, it can be seen that age and all of the characteristics described by percentages are very similar between groups. Renal function is described using median values, and the difference between groups is small in relation to the range within the groups. However, despite using random allocation to groups, systolic blood pressure was 10 units lower in the intervention group, which is an effect size of 0·5 standard deviations between groups. Readers will need to make an expert decision or rely on secondary analyses to decide whether this difference could have biased the final conclusions.

In some studies, information such as age may be best described as a distribution, such as numbers in particular age bands, especially when the data are not normally distributed. In describing data as a mean value, participants with much younger or older ages tend to balance one another, although the standard deviation will give some information of the spread of the data. By giving readers information of the spread of your data, for example the range or standard deviation, you give them sufficient information to judge differences between groups in terms of their clinical importance, which is what they need to do. A *P* value does not help in this. Statistics such as the standard error or a 95% confidence interval, which are measures of precision, are also inappropriate for this purpose. The use of these statistics in tables of baseline characteristics in the literature is common but nevertheless does not provide the information that is required.

If you are reporting the baseline characteristics of the participants enrolled in a randomised controlled trial, this is

Table 3.3 Example of reporting baseline characteristics.

Clinical characteristics of patients randomised to usual care or nurse intervention. Values are numbers (percentages) unless stated otherwise[2]

	Usual care (n = 81)	Nurse intervention (n = 84)
Mean (SD) age (years)	75·6 (7·9)	74·4 (8·6)
Male	44 (51)	54 (64)
Living alone	38 (47)	37 (44)
Social services required	28 (35)	28 (33)
Other medical problems		
angina	40 (49)	38 (45)
past myocardial infarction	41 (51)	46 (55)
diabetes mellitus	15 (19)	15 (18)
chronic lung disease	18 (22)	23 (27)
hypertension	42 (52)	36 (43)
atrial fibrillation	24 (30)	29 (35)
valve disease	12 (15)	15 (18)
past admission for chronic heart failure	36 (44)	27 (32)
New York Heart Association class at admission		
II	16 (20)	19 (23)
III	33 (42)	28 (34)
IV	30 (38)	36 (43)
Degree of left ventricular systolic dysfunction		
mild	10 (13)	18 (22)
moderate	42 (53)	31 (38)
severe	28 (35)	32 (40)
Renal function at admission median (interquartile range)		
plasma urea (mmol/l)	9·7 (6·5–13·9)	8·1 (6·0–10·3)
median (interquartile range)		
plasma cotinine (µmol/l)	116 (90–168)	108 (84–132)
Mean (SD) blood pressure (mmHg)		
systolic	126·1 (21·4)	116 (19·5)
diastolic	70·1 (12·0)	68·4 (10·2)

not a time for significance testing. Hopefully, you did not conduct the study with the purpose of testing whether the baseline characteristics of your participants, who were randomised to study groups, were significantly different merely by chance.[16]

Randomised controlled trials

If you are reporting the results of a randomised controlled trial, you will be required to follow the CONSORT guidelines that are available on the world wide web (www[1]) and have been published widely.[17,18] The guidelines, which were established by an international panel of researchers, statisticians, and epidemiologists, comprise a comprehensive checklist of 22 requirements to help you report the results of your trial fully and accurately. The checklist is shown in Chapter 2. In following the guidelines, you will need to include a flow chart to show how you recruited your sample and how many people were lost at various points in the progression of the study.

If you are reporting the results from a randomised controlled trial, it is important not to submit them as a short report.[19] Short reports are commonly 500–600 words with one table or figure, and preclude the adequate reporting of the study methods that the CONSORT statement was designed to achieve. Even if you are eager to fast track your paper and consider that a short report is more likely to be published and published quickly, do not be tempted to go down this pathway. Many healthcare guidelines are based on systematic reviews or randomised trials. Because you cannot include sufficient information about your methods in a short report, your study will not fulfil the criteria for inclusion in systematic reviews that are fundamental for translating research results into clinical practice.

Case–control studies

In case–control studies, it is important not to report exposures in the case and control groups as percentages or to report mean exposure levels in tables of baseline characteristics. Because these proportions will vary according to the sampling criteria rather than with the prevalence in the general population, they have no inherent epidemiological interpretation and they cannot be compared between studies (www[2]). It is much more valuable if the results are presented as the level of risk that is associated with an exposure, for example as odds ratios. The frequencies of exposed and unexposed cases and controls can then be presented in tables along with the odds ratios but only for the purpose of making the derivation of the statistics transparent to the reader and not for making comparisons with other studies.

Interpretation of results

> *Religion is always right. Religion solves every problem and thereby abolishes problems from the universe... Science is the very opposite. Science is always wrong. It never solves a problem without raising ten others.*

> George Bernard Shaw (in an after-dinner toast to Albert Einstein, 1930)

Always try to present your results in an objective and dispassionate way. Never be tempted to overinterpret your findings, no matter how passionately you believe in your hypothesis and no matter how desperately you want it to be proved. It is much better to limit yourself to describing exactly what you found. For example do not say, *There was an extremely high incidence of disease in the study population.* This is a highly emotive and subjective statement. It is better to present straight facts such as, *The incidence of disease was higher than has been measured previously.* If you need to shout about your results, it is best to do so in private.

You must never state that there was a difference between your study groups when the P value is greater than 0·05. An important concept is that differences between groups that are almost significant, such as those with a P value between 0·051 and 0·1, are not significant. Similarly, you must refrain from making statements such as, *The active group had a larger change from baseline than the control group, although the difference did not reach statistical significance.* These contradictions are confusing in that they suggest that there was a difference between groups although there wasn't. Basically, there is a statistically significant difference between groups or there isn't.

In limiting the interpretation of your results, you should also only extrapolate your findings to participants who are within the range of your study sample. For example, if you found that a treatment was effective but you only enrolled young adult men, you should not suggest that it is an appropriate treatment for the same condition in children, in women, or in older men. Also, never extend your interpretation beyond the bounds of your data. If you have created a regression model for predicting lung volumes from a sample of adults with heights between 140 and 180 cm, do not suggest that your algorithm can be used for shorter or taller people by extending the regression line beyond your study bounds.

The fallout from overinterpreting data can be far reaching. In 2000, a letter to the *BMJ* claimed that a decline in teenage smoking was related to a rise in mobile phone ownership.[20] This finding received much media attention, although the methodologists remained unconvinced. The study design was the weakest type (an ecological analysis) and the result was declared a sad misuse of numbers with the phrase "breathtaking in its inaccuracy"[21] probably justified. Such overinterpretations of results do nothing to further the cause of science, which should always be a considered and dedicated search for the truth.

A *P* value, which is crucial to the way in which we interpret research results, is merely the probability that a result has arisen by chance. The smaller the *P* value the more untenable the null hypothesis.[22] However, it is important to be very careful about the interpretation of *P* values and not to confuse effect size with study size. In studies with a large sample size, small and clinically unimportant differences between groups will become statistically significant simply because the 95% confidence intervals are narrow, precise estimates. This may be good or bad news depending on the purpose of the study.

Basically, it's up to you to interpret your *P* values in terms of the study size, the outcomes measured, and the clinical or public health importance of the results. In measuring the effects of parental smoking on the respiratory health of children, it has been important to conduct very large studies to show that small odds ratios of 1·2 or 1·3 are statistically significant. Although this risk is small, it is important in population terms because rates of exposure to parental smoking are frequently as high as 40% of the population and therefore the absolute number of children in the population who have symptoms as a result of exposure is large. If only a small per cent of children were exposed, a small odds ratio for an outcome that does not have significant clinical implications would indicate that the exposure was of negligible importance to public health. On the other hand, large and clinically important effects may not reach statistical significance in studies with a small sample size.

It is always difficult to interpret results that are on the border of significance but, in doing so, try to be conservative in interpreting the P value and try not to err on the side of over-interpretation. Sometimes it is reasonable to say that a P value between 0·05 and 0·08 is "approaching significance". For example, it may be a fair interpretation of your data to report that, *The difference between the groups would normally be considered to be clinically important but, because of the small sample size, did not reach statistical significance.* In interpreting marginal P values, much depends on the size of the difference between the groups and the size of the study sample. If there was a clinically important difference between the groups but the sample size was small, a marginal P value would suggest that a type II error had occurred and that a larger, more definitive study was warranted. However, if the sample size was large and the difference between groups was small, a marginal P value should probably be ignored. The correct interpretation is always the conservative interpretation and depends entirely on the specific situation.

Finally, do not labour your results by repeating figures or P values in the text that you have already listed in a table. For example, you do not need to report that *A high body mass index was associated with an increased prevalence of shortness of breath ($P = 0·004$).* However you will need to include the P value in the abstract.

Golden rules for reporting numbers

> *The first principle is that you must not fool yourself, and you're the easiest person to fool.*
>
> Richard Feynman, 1992

There are some very good guidelines for reporting numbers.[23] These guidelines, which are summarised in Table 3.4, have the same quirkiness as rules of grammar and must be similarly respected. In essence, most numbers are reported as digits except in some special circumstances.

Table 3.4 Golden rules for reporting numbers.

Rule	Correct expression
Numbers less than 10 are words.	In the study group, eight participants underwent the intervention.
Numbers 10 or more are numbers.	There were 120 participants in the study.
Words not numbers begin a sentence.	Twenty per cent of participants had diabetes.
Be consistent in lists of numbers.	In the sample, 15 boys and 4 girls had diabetes.
Numbers less than 1 begin with a zero.	The *P* value was 0·013.
Do not use a space between a number and its per cent sign.	In total, 35% of participants had diabetes.
Use one space between a number and its unit.	The mean height of the group was 170 cm.
Report percentages to only one decimal place if the sample size is larger than 100.	In our sample of 212 children, 10·4% had diabetes.
Do not use decimal places if the sample size is less than 100.	In our sample of 44 children, 10% had diabetes.
Do not use percentages if the sample size is less than 20.	In our sample of 18 children, two had diabetes.
Do not imply greater precision than your measurement instrument.	Only use one decimal place more than the basic unit of measurement when reporting statistics (means, medians, standard deviations, 95% confidence interval, interquartile ranges, etc.)
For ranges use "to" or a comma but not "–" to avoid confusion with a minus sign and use the same number of decimal places as the summary statistic.	The mean height was 162 cm (95% CI 156 to 168). The mean height was 162 cm (95% CI 156, 168). The median value was 0·5 mm (interquartile range −0·08 to 0·7). The range of heights was 145 to 170 cm.
Rules for data numbers do not apply to citations to the literature.	The page range was 145–70.

In summarising your data, try not to imply more precision than your sample size provides. If you have more than 100 participants in a study group, it is probably OK to report percentages with just one decimal point. However, if you have fewer than 50 participants in the group, then each participant will represent more than 2% of the sample. In this case, it is best to use whole percentages only. If the sample size is fewer than 20 and each participant constitutes more than 5% of the sample, the use of whole numbers is more honest. Similarly, report results with only the same number of decimal places as the measurement itself or perhaps one extra decimal place that is reasonable for a summary statistic. There is no point in implying a precision that does not exist.

Tables

As yet a child, nor yet fool to fame
I lisp'd in numbers, for the numbers came.

Alexander Pope (1688–1744)

Tables are invaluable for presenting numerical results but should not be too large. If many rows or columns are being presented, it is a good idea to consider dividing the table into two. It is also important to keep tables as simple and uncluttered as possible. Row and column headings should be brief but sufficiently explanatory. Standard abbreviations of units of measurements should be added in parentheses.

Take a look in any journal and you will see that published tables do not have multiple borders and grids. Before you create a table, it is a good idea to review the tables in the journal to which you will submit your paper and replicate the style using the border facility of your software package sparingly and appropriately. Fancy borders, shading, and multiple grids are both distracting and unnecessary. Do not be tempted to use them just because you can. In the majority of journals, scientific tables have few horizontal rules and no vertical rules as shown in Table 3.5. You should format your tables in this way with sufficient white space to separate the rows and columns.

The information that you put in the rows and the columns can also be critical. Most people like to read from left to right. Thus, groups that are represented by columns and outcome variables that are shown in rows tend to work well because differences between the groups appear across the page. This

Table 3.5 Example of a scientific table.

Multivariate logistic regression for incident self-reported symptoms of anxiety or depression at year 9. Values are numbers (percentages) unless otherwise stated[24]

	Incident symptoms of anxiety or depression at year 9 (n = 116)	Total (n = 1746)	Adjusted odds ratio (95% CI)	P value
Victimised at baseline				
not bullied in year 8	28 (24.1)	680 (38.9)	1.00	
bullied at one time in year 8	42 (36.2)	575 (32.9)	1.49 (0.88 to 2.54)	0.130
bullied at both times in year 8	46 (39.7)	491 (28.1)	2.03 (1.14 to 3.64)	0.019
Availability of attachments at baseline				
available at both times in year 8	96 (82.8)	1501 (86.0)	1.00	
available at one time in year 8	17 (14.1)	217 (12.4)	1.25 (0.53 to 2.96)	0.594
no available attachments in year 8	3 (2.6)	25 (1.4)	1.97 (0.43 to 9.05)	0.366
Arguments with others at baseline				
none at baseline	31 (26.7)	837 (47.9)	1.00	
with one other at either time	67 (57.8)	798 (45.7)	1.86 (1.05 to 3.30)	0.036
with two or more others at either time	18 (15.5)	104 (6.0)	4.25 (1.82 to 9.94)	0.002
Sex				
male	40 (34.5)	868 (49.7)	1.00	
female	76 (65.5)	878 (50.3)	1.86 (1.02 to 3.40)	0.044
Family structure				
intact family	86 (74.1)	1422 (81.4)	1.00	
separated, divorced, other	30 (25.9)	324 (18.6)	1.47 (0.9 to 2.4)	0.116

makes the interpretation of your data much easier than when the table is organised the other way around. In the table that was shown in Table 3.3, the differences between groups could be easily compared column wise.

As recommended, Table 3.5 also contains the group numbers. In this case the numbers are included in the column titles but they could also be presented as the first line of the table. Inclusion of sample or group sizes helps readers to interpret the data correctly and calculate other statistics that may be of interest to them. It is not a good idea to include sample or group sizes at the base of a table. Table 3.5 is constructed so that it is clear how the summary statistics have been computed and which variables are significant predictors of anxiety or depression. The meanings of "year 8" as the second year of secondary school and "year 9" as 12 months later are defined in the Methods section of the paper.

It is better not to present the same data in both a figure and a table, and never to repeat data from figures or tables in the text. Readers do not want to be given the same information in multiple formats. Indeed, readers may get confused if a percentage of 54·7% in the table is repeated as 55% in the text. Life is too short to spend it trying to decode mystery numbers. It is best to just give the results once, check that they are correct and use a format that gets your message across clearly in one go.

Each table needs a title that tells the reader how to interpret the data. It is much better to have an inclusive title and detailed row and column descriptors than to put the essential information into footnotes, which should be avoided as far as possible. Readers will not want to search the text, the title, and the row and the column headings of the table before finally going to footnotes to find the information that they need before they can interpret your findings. Finally, tables should be submitted on separate pages and not incorporated into the text. It is common practice to print tables one to a page and include them at the end of the manuscript.

Figures and graphics

> *Art does not reproduce what we see; rather, it makes us see.*

> Paul Klee (1879–1940)

Figures and graphs are essential for conveying results in a clear way. A cryptic approach is to show your most important findings as a figure, but only as long as the figure does not take up much more space than reporting the data would. For this reason, some journals prefer tables to bar charts. The figure in which you present your main results should be totally self-explanatory and have a bold, stand-alone quality. A good figure tells the story in a single grab and stays in a reader's mind. Such figures are often taken up by other researchers in their talks to wider audiences and thus help to promote your work. As such, the detail has to be balanced against simplicity.

Figures that you use in talks to colleagues are often too simplified for a journal article in which all of the details must be included in the absence of any accompanying oral explanations. However, figures with too much detail become complicated and difficult to understand when the message gets lost in the graphics and the explanations. The symbols, abbreviations, hatching, line types, and bars must all be very clear and must be explained in detail without cluttering the picture. Also, the figure legend should be comprehensive so that the figure can be fully understood without recourse to reading explanatory text in the results section.

Figures 3.4 and 3.5 show figures that explain the results easily and, as such, add value to their papers. Figure 3.4 shows the magnitude in difference between groups that takes a little longer to work out from the results and statistics presented. Figure 3.5 tells the story almost without having to read the journal article.

Pie charts, which are often useful in oral presentations, have few applications in published journal articles. They are space greedy, the information cannot usually be used to provide an accurate comparison of results between groups, and the numbers are usually better accommodated in a table or bar graph, which takes less space.

When creating a figure, always shrink the printed copy down to the size that it will be in the final copy of the journal and then examine it for legibility. Your work may have to survive a massive reduction during the publication process. Labels that are very readable on an A4 sheet often lose clarity when shrunk into a much smaller format. The most readable figures have large legends and axes descriptors, and use hatching and markings that discriminate clearly between groups. The line

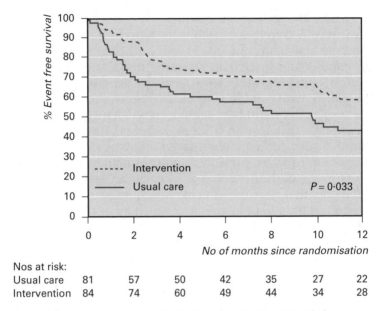

Figure 3.4 Time to first event (death from any cause or hospital admission for heart failure) in usual care and nurse intervention groups.[2]

and hatch details should be substantial enough so that the finished product is suitable for publication, but not too thick so that they cannot be easily interpreted. Fine shades of grey or different colours that look sophisticated in A4 size or in a graph for an audiovisual presentation can look amazingly similar when reduced for publication in black and white.

It is important to try and resist being carried away into the world of computer-generated graphics. Figures should be simple to interpret, uncluttered, and free of extra lines, text, dimensions, and other gimmicks. Never be tempted to use three-dimensional "box" histograms rather than two dimensional histograms. Such histograms are best left as marketing tools because the third dimension has no meaning when presenting scientific results and can create false impressions. The third dimension is not only distracting and meaningless but can prevent readers from being able to interpret the results by comparing the degree of overlap between the 95% confidence intervals. Multidimensional histograms are occasionally used to depict the interactive

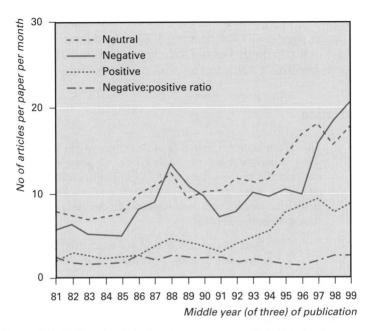

Figure 3.5 Stories about doctors in newspapers (Daily Telegraph, Guardian, and Daily Mail). Three-year rolling means of neutral, negative, and positive articles per paper per month, and the ratio of negative to positive articles.[25]

effects of two factors on an outcome variable and can be useful in oral presentations. However, the relationship can always be explained more precisely in a paper by presenting information from a multivariate model about the absolute size of the interactive effect and whether it is statistically significant.

Photographs, micrographs, and patient records are often essential for explaining the results. These visual aids should always maintain the anonymity of the patient. Many graphics will need to be professionally produced so that any subtle nuances of colour are not lost in the translation to black and white publishing. Some journals will publish coloured photographic images but this is usually at a significant cost to the authors. For most graphics, a scale calibration is needed to interpret the magnitude of the picture and for the comparison of different images.

As with tables, figures should be printed on separate pages and included at the end of the manuscript. Unlike tables, the figure titles, or legends as they are known, are usually listed on a separate page under the heading "Legends to figures". Editors require that you do this rather than copy electronic figures into the text because it helps to facilitate the typesetting processes.

Statistics

> *The experts assure us that farm incomes, on average, are rising. It must be marvellous to sit in an office where you can hear the surf pounding or the flight path overhead and factor in a great winery or booming feedlot with a small rural business or a community on the dole, and get such a reassuring average.*
>
> Jean Kitson (writing on statistics used by politicians, Sydney Morning Herald, 2000)

To avoid bias in your results, it is essential to use the correct statistical tests. The best time to consult a statistician is at an early point in planning your study and not once the data analyses have begun. Statisticians can prevent you from wasting many hours in analysing data in the wrong way and reaching conclusions that are not justified. A statistician can also help to guide you through the processes of dividing your data into outcome or explanatory variables, framing analyses to answer your study questions, choosing the correct statistical test to use, and interpreting the results.

In describing the way in which your data are distributed, you must use the correct measures of central tendency. If the data are normally distributed, the mean is the number to use, but if your data are not normally distributed, the mean will largely underestimate or overestimate the centre of the data depending on the direction of skewness and the standard deviation will be a very inaccurate measure of spread.[14] In this case, always use the median and the interquartile range. In figures and tables, you must always explain whether you are using the standard deviation (SD) as a measure of spread, or the standard error (SE) or 95% confidence intervals as a measure of precision. In general, standard deviations are the correct measurement to describe baseline characteristics, and confidence intervals are the correct measurement to describe precision and assess differences between study groups. It is

Table 3.6 Statistical definitions for central tendency, spread and precision.

	Definitions
Central tendency	
Mean (average)	Measure of the centre of the data Mean = $(\Sigma x/n)$
Median (centre)	The point at which half the measurements lie below and half lie above. Calculated by ranking measurements in order. Median = observation at the middle of the ranked data
Spread	
Standard deviation (SD)	95% of the measurements lie within two standard deviations above and below the mean SD = $\sqrt{\text{variance}}$ Variance = $\Sigma (x_i - \bar{x})^2/n - 1$
Range	Lowest and highest value Calculate by ranking measurements in order
Interquartile range	Range of 25th to 75th percentiles Calculate by ranking measurements in order
Precision	
Standard error (SE)	Estimate of the accuracy of the calculated mean value SE = $SD/\sqrt{n}$
95% confidence interval (CI)	Interval in which we are 95% certain that the "true" mean lies 95% CI = mean $\pm (SE \times 1\cdot96)$

important always to use the abbreviation SD, SE, or CI to define which statistic you are presenting and to avoid using an ambiguous ± or +/– sign. The definitions of some commonly used statistical terms are shown in Table 3.6.

Many researchers choose to use the standard error either as a measure of distribution or as an error bar in figures. However, the standard error is not a descriptive statistic and must not be used as such. Because the standard error is smaller than the standard deviation and approximately half the size of the 95% confidence interval, it suggests that there is much less variability and much more precision than actually exists.

The standard error has no intuitive meaning in making comparisons between groups whereas 95% confidence intervals are an ideal statistic for this purpose.[26]

Journal policies on quoting P values vary widely but, if in doubt, always quote P values exactly. In tables, put $P = 0.043$ not $P < 0.05$, and use $P = 0.13$ not "NS" for indicating a lack of statistical significance. This gives your readers the opportunity to evaluate the magnitude of the P value in relation to the size of your study and the difference between groups that you found. Describing the P value as "NS" or "$P > 0.05$" can be misleading if the actual value is marginal, say 0.07, but the difference between groups is clinically important. Giving the exact value allows readers to make their own judgements about whether it is possible that a type I or type II error has occurred.

Many journals try to keep P values to a minimum. It is certainly a good idea to reserve P values and significance testing for only what you absolutely need to test. This will exclude the significance testing of baseline characteristics in randomised controlled trials. It will also exclude testing for differences between groups when the 95% confidence intervals tell the whole story. The question of whether you should test hypotheses that were not formed prior to undertaking the study is contentious. One golden rule is never to test a hypothesis that does not have biological plausibility. However, new ideas emerge all the time, and the use of existing data sets to explore new hypotheses makes lots of sense if the study design is appropriate for the question being asked. In clinical trials in particular, the need to reduce type I errors has to be balanced with the much more serious problem of avoiding type II errors.[27] The guidelines for the analysis of data from clinical trials[28] should be adhered to at all times.

Multivariate analyses

> *Just as word processing does not ensure better writing, multivariate analyses do not ensure better analyses.*
>
> Kenneth Rothman (www[2])

It is wonderful that, with the burst in new technology and in "click and point" software, multivariate analyses are now accessible to all researchers. However, they should not be misused or abused. Multivariate analyses should never be undertaken until all the univariate and bivariate analyses are evaluated, understood, and tabulated. For example, if you are using logistic regression to measure the association between two exposure variables and an outcome variable, you first need to measure the relation of each exposure to the outcome independently, and the relation between the two exposures. Contingency tables are ideal for this. Until you have a good working knowledge of these three relationships, it may be very difficult to interpret the results of your multivariate model.

It is important to convey results from multivariate analyses in a way that they can be understood, accessed, and compared with the results from previous studies. It is also important that these complex analyses have some degree of transparency to the reader. If you are presenting the results of a one-way or two-way analysis of variance, the mean values and standard deviations in each of the groups or the adjusted mean values should be presented, in addition to the regression equation or the analysis of variance statistics.

Always include adequate summary and subgroup statistics. For example, the β coefficients from logistic regression analyses can be translated into odds ratios, adjusted mean values can be calculated from multiple regression coefficients, or number needed to treat can easily be calculated from between-group differences. This transparency allows the reader to judge the magnitude of the differences between groups and to make comparisons with other studies. It is never helpful to report the results of complex mathematical procedures that cannot be back-translated into an effect size, or to report mathematically complex analyses that are difficult to translate into intuitive results.

Discussion

Say what your findings mean, not what you would like them to mean or think they ought to mean.

JS Lilleyman[29]

The discussion section of your paper should reiterate your main findings but in the context of furthering knowledge or impacting on patient care, public health policy, or future research. This is the time to be honest about any limitations of your study, to explain how your findings fit in with established knowledge, and to explain any inconsistencies. In science, we are continually trying to chip away at parts of a very large jigsaw. The discussion section gives you an opportunity to explain which part of the jigsaw you have put in place.

The discussion can be the most daunting section of a paper to write. If you have a broad knowledge of the literature and of the various opinions in your research field, it can be hard to limit yourself only to the parts that are particularly relevant to your paper. A good trick is to make notes as you analyse your results and read the literature. Jotting down the major ideas that you will need to discuss as they come to mind will help you to organise your discussion section. Also, make notes about which literature supports your findings and which is at odds with your results as you progress. These concept ideas often translate into topic sentences and help to keep each paragraph in focus. The paragraphs can then be ordered from the most to the least important topics. This will help to create a discussion that flows naturally and sensibly.

Figure 3.6 shows a template for writing the discussion section. Paragraph 1 should be a brief summary of what you really found and why it was important. You can restate the aim in more general terms, but do not be tempted to restate the results exactly as in the results section. Good phrases to begin with are, *The results from this study showed that ...; Our results indicate that ...; The purpose of this study was to ... and we found that ...*, etc. This paragraph should focus on the big picture of what your results are really all about. Be bold, explain precisely what you have found, and explain how it will add to current knowledge or change health care.

The second paragraph should address the strengths and limitations of your study design and methods. Honesty is the best policy here. No research is ever perfect and you do not need to be unnecessarily negative about what you have done. However, be honest about how chance, bias, or confounding may have influenced your results, how you minimised this possibility, and how your research is better than what has gone before. Although many readers like to find this information in the second paragraph, it can also be placed later in the section.

The middle paragraphs should explain how your results agree or disagree with other studies and with other related

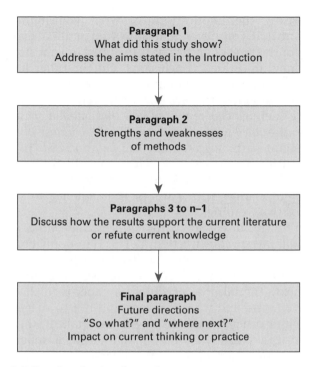

Figure 3.6 Template for the discussion.

theories. Do not be tempted to discuss all the journal articles in every remotely related field. Your readers will only want to know how your findings relate to results from other scientifically valid studies. In this, it is best to confine yourself to discussing the work in your field that is highly relevant and reputable. If you have reached a different conclusion from other researchers who have conducted similar studies, try to explain why you think this has happened. Your references to the literature need to be both focused and brief.

The last paragraph should be an exciting summary of the implications of your findings. The "so what?" of your research needs to be very clear here. The best discussion sections end on a high note with a bit of impact to make a special point. This is a time when you can extend your thinking a little without overstating the implications. There is a fine balance between rhetoric, "spin", and reasonable speculation.[30,31] In summarising the implications of what you found, it is important that you never generalise your results beyond the bounds of the type of participants included in your study, and never draw unjustified conclusions. On the other hand, do not be too tentative if you found a strong association between the exposure and outcomes that you were investigating. A sentence such as, *Our results suggest that vitamin consumption could be associated with a decreased risk of respiratory illness*, has two hesitant parts: *suggest* and *could be associated*. To replace *suggest* with *show* or *could be* with *is* would be firmer but, unless you have conducted a definitive study, it is probably best not to change both parts of the sentence to stronger, more positive wordings.

Never finish a discussion with, *Further studies are needed ...* or *We are now investigating whether ...*. This is not only boring but it is presumptuous to tell your readers what research you consider that they should do, or what you are thinking of doing next. The purpose of writing a paper is to show what you have found and what it means and not to suggest what work you or other researchers might undertake in the future. By writing a clear "so what?", you create a much more interesting and informative end to a paper.

Box 3.4 shows the final paragraphs of the discussion from two studies that produced very similar findings: that people who live in homes with damp or mould have a higher prevalence of respiratory symptoms. The first paragraph ends on a low note in that it suggests that someone else should be prepared to do a better study than the authors have done themselves. The second paragraph ends with impact in suggesting that the results have important implications for public health. Given the wealth of previous literature in this area, this interpretation was justified.

Box 3.4 Final paragraphs from two discussion sections

1. Further studies are needed in which objective measurements of house dampness, exposure to biological contaminants, and health effects are used in addition to questionnaires, so that the associations found in our study and in other studies can be substantiated or refuted.

2. A considerable body of evidence now exists that supports the contention that dampness and mould in the home is an

important public health issue, not solely for its immediate impact but also for the long-term implications. Poor housing conditions in childhood are associated with higher rates of admission to hospital, and higher morbidity and mortality in adult life. Hopefully, planners, policy makers, and medical practitioners will now plan concerted joint action to eradicate this unacceptable and needless health risk.[32]

Some journal editors suggest that discussion sections should not be finished with statements that recommend specific public health actions (www[2]). For example, you may have conducted a questionnaire study and found that some people who are overweight by medical definitions do not consider themselves to be so. In this case, you cannot conclude that, *Public health weight reduction programmes will be ineffective if this finding is not taken into account*, because your finding does not apply to the majority of the overweight community, and you have not collected any evidence to support this. However, there is a strong case for putting your results in a broad community health perspective and suggesting that, *Interventions to counteract personal perceptions may help to improve the effectiveness of weight loss campaigns*. Provided that you do not overinterpret your finding, this kind of finale leaves the reader in no doubt that your results have some implications that could be used to provide better health care.

Summary guidelines

The discussion should not simply stop. It should come to a definite, clear end.

Mimi Zeiger[4]

Box 3.5 below gives a summary of what each section of your paper should contain. Details of how to choose a title, select the appropriate references, and format your paper are explained in following chapters. Further advice can be obtained from the *BMJ* website (www[3]). If you set out to write a paper based on these summary guidelines, your paper should fall into place nicely from the day that you begin writing and it should become a pleasure for your peers and coauthors to review.

Box 3.5 Construction guidelines

Title

Be short, accurate, and unambiguous
Give your paper a distinct personality
Begin with the subject of the study

Introduction

What is known
What is not known
Why we did this study

Methods

Participants
Measurements
Outcomes and explanatory variables
Statistical methods

Results

Sample characteristics
Univariate analyses
Bivariate analyses
Multivariate analyses

Tables and figures

No more than six tables or figures
Use Table 1 for sample characteristics (no *P* values)
Put most important findings in a figure

Discussion

State what you found
Outline the strengths and limitations of the study
Discuss the relevance to current literature
Outline your implications with a clear "So what?" and "Where now?"

References

All citations must be accurate
Include only the most important, most rigorous, and most recent literature
Quote only published journal articles or books
Never quote "second hand"
Cite only 20–35 references

Formatting

Include the title, author, page numbers, etc. in headers and footers
Start each section on a new page
Format titles and subtitles consistently
Comply with "Instructions to authors"

Acknowledgements

The Smiles, Novalis and Pope quotes have been produced with permission from *Collins Concise Dictionary of Quotations, 3rd edn.* London: Harper Collins, 1998 (p 299, 288, 239 respectively). The Dirac, Thompson, Einstein and Feynman quotes have been produced with permission from Horvitz, LA ed. *The Quotable Scientist.* New York: McGraw-Hill Companies, 2000 (p 24, 26, 4, 8 respectively). The Bernard Shaw quote has been produced with permission from the Society of Authors on behalf of the Bernard Shaw estate. The Klee quote has been produced with permission from the Klee estate. All other referenced quotes have been produced with permission.

Websites

1 Consolidated Standards of Reporting Trials (CONSORT)
   http://www.consort-statement.org/revisedstatement.htm
   Guidelines for reporting randomised controlled trials

2 *Epidemiology*
   http://www.epidem.com
   Feature article by K Rothman 'Writing for epidemiology' in *Epidemiology*, 1998:**9**.

3 *BMJ (British Medical Journal)*
   http://www.bmj.com/advice/index.html
   Advice to authors and contributors on how to prepare papers for submission, including checklists, copyright, defining ethnicity, writing advice, etc.

References

1 Lamott A. *Some instructions on writing and life.* Peterborough: Anchor Books, 1994; pp 21, 22, 25, 184.
2 Blue L, Lang E, McMurray JJV *et al.* Randomised controlled trial of specialist nurse intervention in heart failure. *BMJ* 2001;**323**:715–18.
3 Smith R. Introductions. In: *How to write a paper.* Hall GM, ed. London: BMJ Books, 1994.
4 Zeiger M. The introduction. In: *Essentials of writing biomedical research papers.* Maidenhead: McGraw-Hill, 1991; p 2, 184.
5 Benson JR. Guardianship in research. *Lancet* 2001;**358**:1013.
6 Bauchner J, Sharfstein J. Failure to report ethical approval in child health research: review of published papers. *BMJ* 2001;**323**:318–19.
7 Peat JK, Mellis CM, Williams K, Xuan W. Study design. In: *Health science research. A handbook of quantitative methods.* London: Allen and Unwin, 2001.
8 Editorial. Style matters. Ethnicity, race and culture: guideline for research, audit, and publication. *BMJ* 1996;**312**:1094.
9 Editorial. Describing race, ethnicity, and culture in medical research. *BMJ* 1996;**312**:1054.

10   Moher D, Dulberg CS, Wells GA. Statistical power, sample size, and their reporting in randomised controlled trials. *JAMA* 1994;**272**:122–4.
11   Bradford Hill A. The environment and disease: association or causation? *Proc R Soc Med* 1965;**58**:295–300.
12   Belousova EG, Haby MM, Xuan W, Peat JK. Factors that affect normal lung function in white Australian adults. *Chest* 1997;**112**:1539–46.
13   Faniran S, Peat JK, Woolcock AJ. Persistent cough: is it asthma? *Arch Dis Child* 1998;**79**:411–14.
14   Peat JK, Mellis CM, Williams K, Xuan W. Analysing the data. In: *Health science research. A handbook of quantitative methods.* London: Allen and Unwin, 2001; pp 181–202.
15   Norman J. The results. In: *How to write a paper.* Hall GM, ed. London: BMJ Books, 1997; pp 19–29.
16   Altman DG, Dore CJ. Randomisation and baseline comparisons in clinical trials. *Lancet* 1990;**335**:149–53.
17   Altman DG. Better reporting of randomised controlled trials: the CONSORT statement. *BMJ* 1996;**313**:570–1.
18   Rennie D. How to report randomized controlled trials. The CONSORT statement. *JAMA* 1996;**276**:649.
19   Deeks JJ, Altman DG. Inadequate reporting of controlled trials as short reports. *Lancet* 1998;**352**:1908.
20   Charlton A, Bates C. Decline in teenage smoking with rise in mobile phone ownership. *BMJ* 2000;**321**:1155.
21   Jones T. Smoking and use of mobile phones. Data have been wrongly interpreted. *BMJ* 2001;**322**:616.
22   Altman DG. Hypothesis testing. In: *Practical statistics for medical research.* London: Chapman and Hall, 1996; pp 165–71.
23   Lang TA, Secic M. Rules for presenting numbers in text. In: *How to report statistics.* Philadelphia: American College of Physicians, 1997; pp 339.
24   Bond L, Carlin JB, Thomas L, Rubin K, Patton G. Does bullying cause emotional problems? A prospective study of young teenagers. *BMJ* 2001;**323**:480–4.
25   Ali NY, Lo TYS, Auvache VL, White PD. Bad press for doctors: 21 year survey of three national newspapers. *BMJ* 2001;**323**:782–3.
26   Berry G. Statistical significance and confidence intervals. *Med J Aust* 1986;**144**:618–9.
27   Perneger TV. What's wrong with Bonferroni adjustments. *BMJ* 1998;**316**:1236–8.
28   International conference on harmonisation of technical requirements for registration of pharmaceuticals for human use. Statistical principles for clinical trials. *Stat Med* 1999;**18**:1905–42.
29   Lilleyman JS. How to write a scientific paper – a rough guide to getting published. *Arch Dis Child* 1995;**72**:268–70.
30   Horton R. The rhetoric of research. *BMJ* 1995;**310**:985–7.
31   Junger D. Embrace scientific rhetoric for its power. *BMJ* 1995;**311**:61.
32   Platt SD, Martin CJ, Hunt SM, Lewis CW. Damp housing, mould growth, and symptomatic health state. *BMJ* 1989;**298**:1673–8.

4: Finishing your paper

Writing uses words. There are two things you can do with words – choose them and rearrange them.

Mimi Zeiger[1]

The objectives of this chapter are to understand how to:

- write a short, snappy title
- select and quote references correctly
- maximise the value of the peer review process
- package your paper appropriately
- send your paper to a journal
- store your data and your documentation

Choosing a title

It is because assertive sentence titles declare science to be a product that they are to be deplored. By adhering to the idea of science as a process not product, we risk less and may ultimately achieve more.

JL Rosner[2]

Titles take up only a few words but are of inestimable importance in persuading clinicians and researchers to read your paper. If your title has an impact that attracts readers, then so much the better. The basic function of a title is to describe the content of your paper in a succinct way. Also, in these days of database searching, keywords in the title make your paper immediately accessible to workers in your field. However, titles can also be used as a key tool to give your paper a distinct personality. To this end, your title must be accurate, specific, concise, and informative, must not contain abbreviations, and must never be dull. The essential characteristics of an effective title are shown in Box 4.1.

> **Box 4.1 Characteristics of effective titles**
>
> **Effective titles:**
>
> - identify the main issue of your paper
> - begin with the subject of your paper
> - are accurate, unambiguous, specific, and complete
> - do not contain abbreviations
> - attract readers

Short titles are usually best and, in recognition of this, some journals set a limit on the length. For example, some journals ask that the title does not exceed 10–15 words, whilst other journals ask that the title does not exceed two printed lines or a specified number of characters that includes the white spaces. Journals sometimes have specific requirements for titles. For example, *Archives of Diseases in Childhood* asks that the title does not contain the words *child*, *children* or *childhood* because these are implicit in the journal title. They also ask that the study design such as randomised controlled trial, audit, observational study, etc., is included where appropriate.

When writing your title, do not be afraid of trying to attract readers. Just keep working and working on it until you achieve clarity, brevity, and, most of all, human interest. The media strive towards this as a matter of course. For example, on 18 April 2000, when technology stocks crashed wiping out $37 billion in personal wealth in Australia, the *Daily Telegraph* used the headline *Crash.com* and the *Sydney Morning Herald* used the headline *The big shakeout*. Both headlines were effective but the title "*Crash.com*" was catchier, cleverer, and thus more attractive. In the scientific world, the following two journal articles relating to the human genome were published about the same time:

The sequence of the human genome[3]

Initial sequencing and analysis of the human genome[4]

Although both are concise, the first title is shorter and thus more appealing. Writers can gain important insight from examples such as these.

Attractive titles are always concise and to the point. However, a scan of some medical journals shows that many titles are long and boring, and give the impression of being just another journal article that will be tedious to read. Rambling titles are usually convoluted and will not appeal to your external reviewers or improve your readership. Consider the two titles below:

The effect of parental smoking on the development of asthma and other atopic diseases in children: evidence from a birth cohort study in NSW, Australia

Parental smoking and the development of childhood asthma

The first title is comprehensive and descriptive but contains just too many prepositions and qualifiers. It is also not necessary to say things twice. For example, if you use the word *development*, then the method *cohort study* does not need to be added because development cannot be measured in any other type of study. Both titles convey the same message but the second title begins with the main subject of the study *parental smoking* and encompasses the scope of the paper in a few words. The title is much improved by the deletion of the unimportant and unnecessary words. With vigorous pruning, the title becomes snappy and to the point.

However, one word of warning – you must always be accurate and specific in your choice of words and ensure that you do not extend your title beyond the scope of your paper. For example, a review entitled *Respiratory health of Australians* would be expected to contain a broad scope of information about many subjects relating to respiratory health, including information about infections, allergies, smoking outcomes, asthma, and chronic lung disease in both adults and children. On the other hand, a title such as *Asthma and atopy in Australian children* is more specific and may more accurately describe the scope of the review.

There are some simple tricks for improving titles. Since people began to write papers, titles that begin with *On* have suggested something monumental and enduring.[5] The trend was started by Harvey with *On the circulation of the blood* and Darwin with *On the origin of the species*. Now, many researchers aspire to having at least one *On* paper in their publication list. *Toward* is also a good beginning word. In writing a paper with colleagues about a significant advancement in the perplexing problem of defining asthma in population studies, we came up with the title *Toward a definition of asthma for epidemiology.*[6] We liked this title because we felt that it suggested that we had advanced thinking about how to define asthma. We were delighted when the paper and its title were accepted for publication and five years later had achieved a higher citation rate than the impact factor of the journal (4·7 versus 4·4). Impact factors, which are discussed in Chapter 6, are a method of rating the uptake of information presented in a journal article. A title such as *The relationship between symptoms of asthma and airway hyperresponsiveness: results from a population study of children* to describe the same paper may never have achieved such acclaim. Nevertheless, you can have only so many *On* and *Toward* papers on your resume.

Other factors may influence how a title is written. We used the title *Busselton revisited*[7] to compare prevalence data from two population studies just at the time when the BBC series *Brideshead revisited* was enjoying high television ratings. Fellow researchers loved our title and we were runners-up to receive a prize for the work at a national conference. A long descriptive title such as *Evidence for an increased prevalence of asthma in adults living in Western Australia: results from comparative studies in 1981 and 1992* would never have got us so far. Some examples of memorable titles from the literature are shown in Box 4.2. They are all short and concise but they also have an element of intelligence and/or wit. Some use alliteration or references to literature. It is noteworthy that most have a qualitative subtitle that adds to, rather than detracts from, the subject. When browsing the web or undertaking a literature search, many researchers go in and read papers whose titles attract them. However, we acknowledge that you can enjoy far greater licence when designing titles for annotations, reviews, abstracts, and posters than you can for original journal articles.

Box 4.2 Titles from journal articles that attract attention

Egotism in prestige ratings of Sydney suburbs: where I live is better than you think[8]

Twist and shout: deciding when to X-ray a sprained ankle[9]

Beds, bedroom, bedding and bugs: anything new between the sheets?[10]

Did MONICA really say that?[11]

Refeeding of anorexics: wasteful not wilful[12]

Mental distress and the risk of hip fracture. Do broken hearts lead to broken bones?[13]

Similar, the same or just not different: a guide for deciding whether treatments are clinically equivalent[14]

Dissociation in people who have near-death experiences: out of their bodies or out of their minds?[15]

Are you busy for the next 5 years? Recruitment in the Childhood Asthma Prevention Study[16]

African origin of modern humans in East Asia: a tale of 12,000 Y chromosomes[17]

Losing the battle of the bulge: causes and consequences of increasing obesity[18]

The title of a journal article should have minimal punctuation. That said, for better or worse, punctuated titles have increased in popularity. The number of colons used in titles increased significantly in the *BMJ* and the *Lancet* between 1970 and 1995, but not in the *New England Journal of Medicine*.[19] It is unclear whether authors used colons to appeal to the editors of the first two journals, or whether editors of the *New England Journal of Medicine* removed any colons they found. Writers often use punctuation to add a qualifying subtitle even though subtitles that describe the study design are often unnecessary or can detract from the title's impact. For example, in the title *Risk factors for birth defects in premature babies: a case–control study*, the study design could be removed. While study design is of fundamental importance for any clinical or epidemiological research study, it is better described in the Abstract and the Methods rather than in the title, unless the journal suggests otherwise.

A traditional title tells readers what the journal article is about in an open way and invites them to judge the results by the contents. Three different methods of writing a title are shown in Box 4.3. The classic way of writing a title is to begin with a word that describes the main topic or the independent variable in your analyses. If the paper is submitted to a respiratory journal, either of the first two titles in Box 4.3 would suffice, but for a journal concerned with growth, the third title would be more appropriate. The problem with these types of titles is that they can be boring, especially if they are not short and concise.

Box 4.3 Different ways of writing titles

Titles that give independent variable, dependent variable, and population:

Effect of asthma on linear growth in children
Asthma and linear growth in children
Final height attainment of asthmatic children

Titles that pose a question:

Does asthma reduce linear growth?
Are asthmatic children shorter than non-asthmatic children?

Titles that give the answer to the question:

Asthma is negatively associated with growth in height during adolescence
Linear growth deficit in asthmatic children

There is an increasing tendency to use questions in titles. Questions that reiterate the aim of the paper may attract readers who want to know the answer. However, such titles are frowned on, perhaps because they tend to suggest a positive result and are therefore misleading if the findings are negative. Fashions rarely last and question titles are probably best reserved for abstracts and talks, which can be more immediate and interactive. Journal articles need to be more conservative in the ways in which results are conveyed, and their titles need to withstand the tests of time.

The "assertive sentence title" has grown in popularity but should be avoided at all costs for journal articles. These titles give an answer to the study question and, as such, convey an impression of eternal truth that does not leave room for the possibility of error.[20] Such titles tell the answer to the question and often suggest much larger differences between study groups than was actually found. For example, a height deficit in asthmatic children that was minimal in magnitude and therefore of no clinical importance, but which reached statistical significance because of a large sample size, should not be reported under either of the last two titles shown in Box 4.3. Whilst these titles work well to attract attention amongst the poster rows at a conference, they should certainly not be used to report study results in a journal article. In fact, some journals such as the *New England Journal of Medicine* request that declarative titles are not used.

All too often, assertive sentence titles cannot be proved beyond reasonable doubt or cannot be entirely substantiated. Bold conclusions about research results in the title are often reported much more tentatively in the article itself and inevitably tend to misinform the reader. It is also a problem when a title turns out to be an error but remains embedded in the literature forever. Inevitably, assertive sentence titles trivialise reports from scientific studies by reducing them to one-liners when the data may ultimately prove to be of more value than the single advertised conclusion.[20]

In a survey of assertive sentence titles, 24 journal articles that used the verb *prevents* did not always describe a treatment that prevented a clinical condition.[21] Despite the misleading nature of such titles, journal editors often find them useful for attracting readers because they suggest a clear take-home message.[22,23] However, this is not desirable when the message is inaccurate, overstated, or unqualified. In recognition of this, the occasional researcher who has used the assertive sentence title has been taken to task. The authors of a journal article entitled *Improved survival for patients with acute myelogenous leukemia* were criticised for making such a bold, optimistic conclusion from the results of a single institution pilot study.[23] The implied statement in the title about the efficacy of a new treatment could only have been reached using a large, multicentre, randomised controlled trial and, even then, an assertive sentence title should not be used.

Above all else, a title must be factually correct. When we were working with colleagues on a paper, the title *Increasing weight is a risk factor for asthma in childhood* was initially suggested. The problem with this title is that it suggests that gaining weight rather than being overweight is a risk factor for asthma. Eventually, we agreed on the title *Overweight children and the risk of asthma*. In this way, the subject of the paper was encompassed in the first two words *overweight children*, and the keywords *overweight*, *risk* and *asthma* were all included so that other authors would be able to retrieve the article easily when searching reference databases. Most importantly, the results were relegated to the results section where they belonged and our final title was shorter, concise, and therefore more attractive.

In the end, it is up to you to devise the best title that you can for your paper. In this, try and work towards a title that is short, informative, attractive, and factually correct. However, try not to be disappointed if your paper is accepted for publication and the title is ultimately rewritten by the journal editors.

Title page

Scientific writers are terrified of journalism and, desperately anxious to avoid any hint of sensationalism or hyperbole, veer too far in the direction of tedious obscurity.

JS Lilleyman[24]

Once the authors and title are decided, it is exciting to create a title page for your paper to give it a formal look. Most journals specify the requirements for the title page in their *Instructions to Authors* and these will vary according to journal requirements. The title page usually has the title at the top and the authors clearly listed below. All authors must be listed regardless of how many there are. Many journals limit the number of authors and request that if there are more than 12, other names must appear in a footnote. If more than 12 authors are listed for a multicentre trial or more than eight from a single institution, each author may be required to sign a statement attesting that they fulfil the authorship criteria of the ICMJE (www[1]). Authors should be listed with their full names, highest academic degree, title/s, position, and address. You should also include the name of the department and institution where the work was undertaken, the institutional affiliation and full contact details of yourself as the first author. Finally, add a direct telephone number and facsimile number with their international dialling codes and the email address from which reprints should be requested. You must also acknowledge any grant support either on the title page or in the acknowledgements section.

The title page should also include a running title, which is the title abbreviated to the number of letter spaces requested by the journal, usually 30–40 including white spaces. This title will appear in the header or footer of the journal pages other than on the title page. Finally, select 3–10 key words or short phrases to add to the bottom of the title or abstract page. Standard terms should be selected from the Medical Subject Headings (MeSH), which can be found at the MEDLINE® website (www[2]) or in the printed *Index Medicus* held by medical libraries. This will help to ensure that your paper is indexed correctly in the electronic databases and can be found easily by other researchers. Journals may have slight variations in the information that they require on the title page, so always check in the *Instructions to Authors*.

References and citations

After all, the ultimate goal of all research is not objectivity, but truth.

Helene Deutsch (1884–1982, www.bartelby.com)

The citation section of a paper is important for giving credit to the ideas and work of other scientists. In finding the references that you need, you can use the web to search MEDLINE® via PubMed® (www[3]) or you can use other websites to find links to further references and to netprints (www[4–8]). If you are quoting a method, a sentence, an idea, or some results published by another researcher, then you must cite the original source. Using other researchers' ideas or any parts of their writing as your own is a serious offence known as plagiarism.

When you are writing a journal article, you need to cite only the most valid, most important, and most recent literature. Ideally, you conducted a full literature search when the study was planned and you have updated it as the study progressed.

If you are organised, you will have your references stored in an electronic database such as Endnote® or Reference Manager® (www[9]). This will allow you to format a bibliography in a fraction of the time that it takes to do it manually. In addition, your paper copies will be filed in alphabetical order or in an indexed or linked file so that they are readily retrieved. Even better, you will have read all of the original journal articles that you plan to cite. Before you submit your paper with a reference list created using a computer package, check with your editor that the format is acceptable. Some journals prefer to use their own templates.

There is a much greater need to be selective rather than to be inclusive with the references that you quote in your introduction and discussion, which are essentially narrative reviews. It is best to only include references that are published in peer-reviewed journals and to exclude any references to unpublished work or abstracts. It is also best to cite only the data from studies that have been rigorous and provide high quality evidence. By selecting the most rigorous literature, you will raise the standard of your paper. The golden rule for an original article is to cite 20–35 references maximum although some journals set specific limits that may be larger or smaller than this.

In your paper, you will need to cite your references in the style requested by the journal. The citation of references is usually in numerical order throughout your paper with the references listed at the end using Vancouver format (Box 4.4) (www[1]). However, some journals such as *Nature* adhere to their own style. The citation of books and book chapters is usually specific and should be checked with the *Instructions to Authors* (www[10]). Although most journals have moved to Vancouver format, some still retain their own format and most electronic database systems have various style options to allow for this.

Box 4.4 Examples of citations presented in Vancouver format for the reference section

Bhopal R, Rankin J, McColl E, Thomas L, Kaner E, Stacy R, *et al*. The vexed question of authorship: view of researchers in a British medical faculty. *BMJ* 1997;**314**:1009–12.

> Kenyon SL, Taylor DJ, Tarnow-Mordi W, for the ORACLE Collaborative Group. Broad-spectrum antibiotics for preterm, prelabour rupture of fetal membranes: the ORACLE I randomised trial. *Lancet* 2001;**357**:979–988.
>
> von Mutius E. Progression of allergy and asthma through childhood to adolescence. *Thorax* 1996;**51** (Suppl.):S3–S6.
>
> Armon KA, Elliott EJ. Acute gastroenteritis. In: Moyer VA, Elliott EJ, Davis RI *et al.*, eds. *Evidence-based pediatrics and child health*. London: BMJ Books, 2000.

In Vancouver format, the author list must have surnames followed by initials with no full stops and separated by commas. When citing a reference, the first six authors are listed followed by *et al.* The National Library of Medicine (www[3]) lists up to 24 authors before *et al.* is used, whereas Vancouver format requires that only six are listed. The author list is followed by one space and then the title. The title is followed by a full stop, one space, the journal name abbreviated using *Index Medicus* guidelines, one space, the year of publication, a semicolon, the volume, a colon and then the page numbers followed by a full stop. Issue numbers or the dates of volumes are not included. Abbreviated journal names are published each year in the January issue of *Index Medicus* or can be found at the website (www[2]). If you are unsure of the correct abbreviation to use, quote the journal name in full since it is not acceptable to make up your own abbreviation.

The use of an electronic reference management database (www[9]) is an essential tool for any writer. Because most reference manager programs will readily produce reference lists in a variety of styles and formats, it is prudent to invest in using this type of software. In this way, the reference needs only to be entered once, perhaps by downloading from a bibliographic database such as MEDLINE® or PubMed®. You can then add and delete references or reorganise the text in your paper in the knowledge that your software will renumber your references correctly in the final version.

It is essential that you verify that your references are correct. You should never use phrases in your paper or enter citations into your database that you have copied from another paper. Even public databases may have some errors, so always be thorough and obtain a copy of the original article so that you can check that your electronic references are absolutely correct. It is essential to ensure that the article says what other people say it says and check its exact citation details. You can then cite any article liberally in the knowledge that the reference is always correct. Errors in the year of publication, the volume number or the page numbers make it very difficult and very frustrating for fellow researchers who want to retrieve the cited article. High error rates that have been identified in citations, mostly in authors' names and the title,[25] are both unacceptable and easily preventable.

As an author, you are entirely responsible for the accuracy of your references, the details of which will not be checked by the journal or copy editors. Good scientists pay attention to detail in all of their work. Errors in references detract from the quality of your paper and suggest that you may also have lacked attention to detail in collecting and reporting the data. Moreover, quoting second-hand sets up chains of Chinese whispers that perpetuate errors as they are transcribed from one author to the next. As such, these compounding errors will detract from your scientific reputation because your mistake will become public when the *Scientific Citation Index* (see Chapter 6) records your incorrect citations and helps to pinpoint their origin.

When you are writing your paper, always quote the science and not the scientist.[1] Although the names of researchers are quoted extensively in the behavioural sciences, they do not need to be quoted in clinical research. When you cite the work of other researchers, you need to compare your results with their results or say what they found. You should do this without using the authors' names in the text. Rather than writing *Smith* et al. *found that the prevalence of diabetes in 1998 was 8%*, it is much more informative to write, *In a cross-sectional study conducted in 1998, the prevalence of diabetes was 8%*.

If you use some researchers' names and not others, you tend to add a name dropping importance to selective work. Also, the practice ignores the contributions of the coauthors whose names are omitted. It is best not to use names at all but, if you really do want to, then you should use them consistently for all citations throughout. If you really want to cite another research group by name, be convinced that you really need to do this and only cite the head of the research group. Usually, there is a better alternative. That said, on rare occasions it may be important to highlight the work of another group of scientists, for example when you are writing rebuttals to comments made by the reviewers of a grant application.

When you are citing the literature in a paper, always use conservative phrases. Never say *It is widely believed that* ... when you have few recent references to back up the claim, or *Much recent interest has centred around* ... when few people have published on the topic in recent years.[5] Similarly, phrases such as *It has long been known that* ... or *It is generally believed that* ... are best avoided. If there is a substantial body of high level evidence to back up a statement, you probably don't need to write about it at all because it will almost certainly be common knowledge. Many journals allow you to cite narrative reviews, but it is not a good idea to quote the personal opinions of review writers. Limit your paper to facts not opinions.

In most journals, you cannot cite personal communications, unpublished work, or conference abstracts. If the journal does allow the citation of personal communications, you will need to obtain written permission from the person cited and give their title, position, and affiliations. If you want to cite a paper that has been submitted but not yet accepted for publication, you should include a copy of the manuscript of that paper together with your paper when you send it to a journal. If the citation of an informal data source, such as verbal or written information, is acceptable to a journal, and often it is not, then it is cited as follows: R.A. Brown (personal communication, 18 March 2000). Such references appear only in the text and are not included in the reference list. Email communications should be cited as personal communications.

Increasingly, information found on the web may be acceptable for inclusion in some journals and, if so, should follow the standard citation style shown below. All electronic references must give the same information as for a printed source but, because web content and addresses frequently change, web citations must include the retrieval date. An example of a correct web citation is as follows:

> *American Psychological Association. How to cite information from the internet and world wide web.*
>
> www.apastyle.org/elecref.html
> (accessed 19 Nov 2001)

If a website is being included in the text without a citation in the reference list, only the web address is given as in, for example *Information about how to cite reports, magazines, newspaper articles etc can be found at http:/www.windsor.igs.net* Further information on how to cite different sources can be found on the internet (www[11,12]).

Peer review

> *A naturalist's life would be a happy one if he had only to observe and never to write.*
>
> Charles Darwin (1809–1892)

Peer review is the cornerstone of good science but, that said, it is a peculiar process. The peer-review process is inherently fraught with difficulty because you are essentially asking for criticism, although you would, no doubt, prefer praise. To receive praise is a truly wonderful, feel-good experience, but only the criticism can help to improve your paper. Although you need peer review, criticism is hard to take no matter how it is packaged, so take a deep breath, put your feelings aside, and remember that, if your coauthors misinterpret what you have written or find your paper difficult to read, then others will too.

The quality of peer review can vary widely from positive comments, ticks, and slight alterations of wording through to abject, unwarranted criticism and suggestions that your paper requires a complete rethink. Fortunately, the best peer review resides in the middle ground and provides positive suggestions for change and improvement. In planning who to select to peer review your work, it is a great advantage if you have a mentor who is able to provide insight and creativity, and who can help you to negotiate your way through the review process. This is discussed further in Chapter 12. Whatever type of feedback you receive, it will almost certainly be both the most confronting and the most valuable contribution to the development of your paper.

Once your paper is underway, it is time to ask for peer review from either your coauthors or coworkers. This will help to ensure that the methods have been described in detail, that the results are reported accurately, and that the findings are stated clearly and are not overinterpreted. This is vital for upgrading the standard of your paper, both in terms of the science and the presentation. Peer review will help you to develop your ideas, improve the scientific integrity of your results, and produce an eminently more readable paper.

The good news is that, with good writing practice, peer review should not be too painful or too depressing. If you start with a plan in mind, design the paper with a purpose, and write in short, clear sentences, you will create a product that the reviewers will find easy to read and therefore can respond to more easily in an intellectual way. This is important because intellectual contributions are far more valuable to the advancement of papers than comments on grammar and organisation. When papers are badly constructed and poorly written, reviewers tend to concentrate on trying to fix the immediate problems of presentation rather than thinking about the content and the big picture. This, in turn, prompts an endlessly frustrating review-edit-amend roundabout without any major focus on content.

Naturally, it is better if a paper stays on a sensible and planned track from day one rather than being continually pushed and pulled into everyone's different ideas of what shape it should take. Constructing a paper with well-articulated aims from square one tends to focus on content and to ensure that major structural changes are not requested at the end, just when you thought you were finished. If you can achieve this, the whole review process is shorter and more purposeful, and everyone enjoys the rewards of seeing the paper progress quickly towards a publishable document.

By asking for peer review, you are in effect asking colleagues to assist you with the scholarship of your work. This is a system that should be treated with the utmost respect. You should never pass a draft out for review before it is truly ready, that is before it has reached the highest standard to which you can take it. The thoughtlessness of repeatedly handing out ill-prepared documents tends to wear reviewers down. To receive the most valuable feedback, drafts must be at the highest standard that you can possibly achieve before you ask your colleagues for comment. This will ensure that everyone spends their time efficiently because the number of drafts is minimised and the quality of the feedback is maximised.

If it is at all possible, drafts should be circulated serially, that is to one reviewer at a time, and not in parallel, that is to all of your coauthors at once. By incorporating each reviewer's improvements before you pass the document on again, the next reviewer receives the most advanced version of your work and coauthors do not have to duplicate each other's work. Some groups of coauthors find it is very productive to hold miniwriters' groups and brainstorm some ideas together rather than reviewing in isolation. It is important to find a reviewing process that is both efficient and suits the work practices of your authorship team.

Between drafts, you will need to strive to be your own best critic. As well as taking the coauthors' and reviewers' comments on board, you need to continually work on each paragraph so that the topic sentence is accurate and correct, the grammar is flawless, and the sentences have a minimum number of words and flow together nicely. Methods for achieving this are discussed in Chapters 8–11. This should not be an arduous task but rather a rewarding process of finding better ways to package your science, your results, and your ideas. Your paper is ready to circulate only when it gives you pleasure to read.

It is up to you as the first author to decide whether you want verbal, written, or electronic feedback. Written feedback on a paper copy of your draft article is often the optimal way to proceed but this assumes that your reviewer's handwriting is legible! There is an increased move towards electronic feedback using the "track changes" facilities of word processing packages. The problem is that if you send reviewers an electronic copy of your paper to edit on their screen, then you are in effect giving them temporary ownership of the document. Also, it can be difficult to transfer electronic changes to your master document if it has been altered since you gave a copy of it out for review. Always make sure your reviewer knows how to use the system if it is acceptable. With either paper or electronic editing, you will have to ensure that your reviewers understand that you will accept, amend, or reject their suggestions as you see fit and not necessarily accept them all *per se*.

People often discuss how many drafts are needed before a fledgling paper evolves into a well-written paper, with numbers of 20 or 30 often suggested. However, if you think of a draft as a paper in progress that you hand to your coauthors for feedback, these numbers are excessive. It is much more satisfying if your paper takes shape and becomes a pleasure for your coauthors and reviewers to progress in a few drafts. It is also rewarding to find a concise way to tell people what you want them to know. Many researchers find it exciting to turn their fledgling draft into a sensible, well-written, and beautifully presented paper, despite having to endure the problems and politics of the peer-review processes.

Processing feedback

Science is nothing but trained and organised common sense.

Thomas Henry Huxley (1894–1963)

Asking for review, by default, invites suggestions about changing your paper. All reviewers will have their own ideas about how your paper should be written, what the content should be, and how the whole thing should be packaged. Sometimes these ideas will be radically different from your own ideas. This is when good communication skills are needed.

In dealing with peer review, remember that you cannot keep all the people happy all the time. However, as the first author, it is your job to consider all the comments that you receive and to decide carefully which ones to take on board, or not as the case may be. Ideally, the coauthors should have agreed on the aims before you began. It then becomes your job to focus on what the paper is about and to keep it on track from the beginning to the end of the process.

Peer-review comments should always be taken seriously. Having put out requests for review on the content, the grammar, the sentence structures, etc., you should try and accommodate any suggestions. This can be difficult if you have become so bonded with your paper that you are unwilling to make any major changes. If the reviewers are suggesting seemingly daunting changes, it is a good idea to retreat and spend some time thinking through the problems, but do not put your paper on the back burner for too long. Remember that bad news is not so bad if slept upon. There is nearly always a way to improve a manuscript, and making changes will almost always be for the better. Meeting people half way is a good networking skill. If necessary, ask a third party to adjudicate.

Of course, constructive and positive feedback is always easy to deal with and to be grateful for, but, even if you receive negative feedback, it is polite to thank reviewers for their suggestions and deal with them graciously. Reviewing takes time, and fellow colleagues' best efforts at reviewing, like your best efforts at writing, should not be lightly dismissed. It is understandable to feel pressure to publish and to want to submit your paper quickly, but try to be objective and focus on the big picture. All suggestions can lead to improvements in one way or another, and respecting your reviewers' comments will help to foster better collaborative links. On the other hand, being argumentative or dismissive of reviewers' suggestions will be remembered in many ways, and will not help to promote your academic career or your scientific reputation.

Checklists and instructions to authors

> *At all stages of preparation of the paper, go back and check with the instructions to authors and make sure that your manuscript conforms. This seems very obvious but if you wish to publish in the* European Annals of Andrology *do not write your paper to conform with the* Swedish Journal of Androgen Research.
>
> George Hall[26]

The *Instructions to Authors* for each journal can be found on the web (www[10]). Because journals all have different requirements, it is more efficient to write your paper in the correct format to begin with rather than have to alter it later. For example, some journals request that all the results are presented in tables with numbers for everything, including the numerator and denominator of percentages, whereas other journals prefer percentages in the tables or figures for the main results.

In addition to checking your paper against the journal's requirements, it is a good idea at some stage to check the contents of your paper against the type of checklist that is used by reviewers. There are many reviewer checklists available and some journals such as *BMJ* and *JAMA* publish these on their websites (www[13,14]). If your external reviewers are going to use one of these checklists, you should too. A generic compilation of commonly used checklist questions is shown in Box 4.5.

If you are reporting data from a randomised controlled trial, then it must conform to the CONSORT statement[27] (www[15]) as listed in Chapter 2, but different checklists can be used for qualitative studies, statistical reviews, economic evaluations, etc. (www[15]). Checklists that can be used to present results from randomised controlled trials, case–control, cohort, cross-sectional, or ecological studies can be found on the *BMJ* website (www[13]) and the Cochrane Collaboration has standard guidelines for the presentation of systematic reviews (www[16]).

Box 4.5 Checklist questions for reviewers and writers

General

Is the work original?
Is the information important?
Was the study ethical?
Does the work add enough to what is already in the literature?
Is the title accurate and informative?
Does the abstract include the most important results?
Does the paper read well and make sense?
Are the results of interest to the readers of this journal?

Introduction

Is the length of the introduction reasonable?
Does the introduction adequately review the background and state the aims?

Methods

Are the methods well documented and detailed enough?
Are the participants adequately described and their conditions defined?
Was a satisfactory response rate achieved?
Is the equipment used adequately described?
Are the techniques used adequately described and validated?
Were the methods suitable for the study?
Is a calculation of the required sample size given?
Are all statistical methods adequately described and referenced?

Results

Is the description of the results clear and detailed?
Are the results credible, valid, and well presented?
Are the statistical methods appropriate?

(continued)

Are confidence intervals given where necessary?
Are the numbers in the text independent of the numbers in the figures and tables?
Are the stated results supported by the statistical analyses?

Discussion

Is the length of the discussion appropriate?
Does the discussion adequately consider the limitations of the study?
Does the discussion fairly review previous work?
Do the conclusions answer the aims set out in the introduction?
Are the conclusions justified and logical?

Tables and figures

Are the figures of adequate quality?
Are all of the tables and figures necessary?
Do the legends and titles of the tables and figures provide adequate information?

References

Are all of the references relevant?
Do the references fairly represent current knowledge in this field of research?
Is any major literature omitted?
Are there any misquotations or incorrect citations?

Remember that external reviewers are usually asked by editors to rank the quality of your paper. They are often asked whether it is suitable for publication in terms of yes, no, or uncertain, whether publication should be routine or fast track, and whether the quality is excellent, good, fair, or poor. Reviewers are also sometimes asked if the paper should be sent to a biostatistician for expert review and to score attributes such as creativity and originality, scientific importance, study design, interpretation, clarity, and brevity. If you are unsure about the quality of your paper, it may be prudent to devise your own checklist and give it to your internal peer reviewers or coauthors to elicit this type of feedback.

Creating a good impression

Like it or not, first impressions often count a lot – so people could get the wrong idea of what you are all about just by looking at you.

Granville Toogood[28]

People who want to succeed in the heady world of corporate high fliers are very aware of the importance of packaging both themselves and their presentations to impress their peers. There is every reason to adopt this model for your paper. When you submit your paper to a journal, you are in effect sending it out for a job interview. The paper is much more likely to be accepted if it looks smart, is sensible, and fulfils the journal's requirements.

Although creating the correct packaging takes time, it is time well spent. Visually attractive papers are more tempting to readers and organised writing helps to sustain reader interest. Within each section of your paper, you will need clear, concise paragraphs that are easy on the reader's mind and transmit your messages in a very simple way. Once this is achieved, you need to format and organise your paper. Box 4.6 summarises some methods for this. Most journals request that you double-space your document. This naturally creates white space and avoids the walls of text that readers find daunting; it is also essential for the copy editors to mark up your hard copy prior to printing, if it is not being edited on screen. Paying attention to the formatting and organisation has a double advantage. The end result will not only look better but will read better too.

Box 4.6 Organising your paper

Visual appeal

Use ample white space
Number your pages
Put identification information in a header or footer
Start each new section on new page
Write short paragraphs
Left-justify and double-space the text
Avoid hyphenating words between lines
Eliminate orphan lines

Visual topic changes

Use subheadings to divide sections
Use new paragraphs for new topics

Verbal topic changes

Use a new topic sentence to begin each paragraph

Make sure that your front page looks attractive and check it for completeness. To improve readability for your reviewers, left-justify your paper, leaving the right-hand side ragged rather than creating inconsistent and annoying gaps in lines, especially lines with long words. It is also best to ignore the hyphenation option of your word processor that divides words in the most unlikely places. Finally, check your print-preview screens to ensure that no orphan lines are stranded on new pages. Word pruning to shrink the section back is usually preferable but adjusting the margins can also prevent the problem.

Because most journals do not specify a font, you should choose one that reflects the mood that you want your paper to convey. It is best to choose a font that looks serious, traditional, and professional rather than playful or trendy. Fun fonts such as Comic Sans MS are great for talks and may be more interesting to write your drafts and think in, but are not suitable when submitting a paper to a journal. Also, choose a font size that is easily legible. Many reviewers work in less than optimal lighting areas such as aeroplanes, hotel rooms, and even bedrooms. You need to ensure that your paper can maintain its readability under these conditions.

Pay most attention to your tables and figures. For clarity, you will have written your results section so that most of the numbers are in the tables and the explanations are in the text. In presenting numbers, precision is everything. Always check and then double-check both the numbers and the statistics that you present. For example, if you have 18 out of 80 participants who have a disease, then the percentage is 22·5%. It is confusing if percentages imply that the number of participants with a disease is not a whole number. For example, if a percentage of 22·5% is erroneously reported as 22·9%, then we would infer that 18·3 participants had the disease. Miscalculations such as this are confusing and detract from the validity and believability of your results.

Once you feel the manuscript is finished and ready to go, put it away for a week before making a final check of the *Instructions to Authors*. Then find time for one last read to review the content and appraise the appearance. An obsessive-compulsive approach is a mark of a good scientist, and paying attention to the small details can have large benefits in the end. Every little bit of improvement will help to convince your peers that you are a careful and well-organised writer and that your work deserves to be published.

The very last thing that you want to do is send away a paper that looks boring, uninviting, and disorganised. A paper that looks smart on paper sends positive visual messages to your reviewers that you have assembled it with a great deal of thought rather than dispatched in a dispassionate way. An untidy, disorganised paper just begs to be sent back to the writer, perhaps before it has even been read.

Submitting your paper

Most of my successes have come out of failures.

Charles Townes (physicist and Nobel laureate who
codeveloped the laser, 1995)

Once you have chosen the journal and survived the draft processes, checked that your paper is complete, and given it one final appraisal to ensure that it looks good and reads beautifully, you are ready to send your paper to a journal. Never hesitate to give your final draft one last proofread, one last spell check, and one last walk through the checklists and *Instructions to Authors* before you put it into the envelope or press the submit button. Finally, write a covering letter to the editor as shown in Box 4.7. Although only the first author need sign the covering letter, some journals also require all authors to sign a copyright form, which must accompany the covering letter when the paper is submitted.

Box 4.7 Example of a letter to the editor

Dear Editor

Please find enclosed a paper entitled 'Exact statistical methods for presenting data of rare diseases' for consideration for publication in your journal.

The data included in this manuscript have not been published previously and are not under consideration by any other journal. A form with consent to publication signed by the authors is enclosed. All authors have read this final manuscript and have given their approval for the manuscript to be submitted in its present form.

(continued)

I enclose:

- three paper copies of the manuscript
- three copies of the tables and figures
- a labelled disk containing the electronic version.

As the corresponding author, my contact details are shown on the cover page of the manuscript.

Yours sincerely

Although some journals now accept electronic submissions, many journals still require paper communication, especially for the first submission. If you use the electronic method, carefully follow the journal instructions about file formats and how to separate your paper into the separate electronic files that are required for the text, the tables, and the figures. If you do submit your paper electronically, you are likely to receive an automated reply when your paper is received. If electronic submission is not available or you chose not to use it, then package the required number of paper copies in a strong envelope that will survive a national or international journey. If you are enclosing photographs, sandwich them in strong cardboard to prevent them from being dented or folded en route. Also, label them clearly on the reverse with your name and the title of your paper, marking the labels before you attach them to the photos, so that you do not indent the photograph.

Always keep exact electronic and paper copies of the manuscript you submitted to the journal together with the correspondence, figures, photographs etc. You should receive an acknowledgement that your paper has reached the journal editor within one month of sending it and a letter from the editor about the status of your paper within four months. Papers occasionally get lost in the mail and occasionally get lost in the system after they have been officially received by the journal. If you do not receive your letters from the editor, it pays to consider these possibilities.

Archiving and documentation

It is easy to fit the pieces of the puzzle together if you distort their shape but, when you have done so, your success is no proof that you have placed them in their original positions.

Philip Lake (disputing Wegener's theory of continental drift in 1928; 1865–1949)

Once your paper is submitted, the data and all of the documentation surrounding the data analyses should be stored in a durable and appropriately referenced form. Wherever possible, the original data in the form of questionnaires, data collection sheets, CDs, medical records, etc. should be safely retained in the department or unit where they were generated. Data should be held safely for as long as readers of publications might reasonably expect to be able to raise questions that require reference to them. Some research funding bodies stipulate that this should be at least five years, others state 10 years. Before you discard your data or the documentation of your data analyses, you must be certain that you are not contravening the policies of either your institution or your funding bodies.

All references to where the data are held and how it is archived should be logged in a study handbook that is freely available to all stakeholders and research staff who have been involved in the study.[29] The handbook should include all details of the names and locations of electronic data files and databases, data recodes and transformations, and data analyses programs and output. Although individual researchers may hold copies or subsets of the data, a complete data set free of errors and updated with all corrections must be archived and safely stored at all times. In this way, anyone can repeat your analyses or use the data set to answer new questions as they arise.

Acknowledgements

The Huxley quote has been produced with permission from *Collins Concise Dictionary of Quotations, 3rd edn.* London: Harper Collins, 1998 (p 168). The Townes and Lake quotes have been produced with permission from Horvitz, LA ed. *The Quotable Scientist.* New York: McGraw-Hill Companies, 2000 (p 27, 154 respectively). All other referenced quotes have been produced with permission.

Websites

1 International Committee of Medical Journal Editors (ICMJE)
   http://www.icmje.org
   Uniform requirements that provide instructions to authors on how to
   prepare manuscripts to submit to biomedical journals including links to
   sites about sponsorship, authorship and accountability

2 *Index Medicus* (United States National Library of Medicine)
   http://www.nlm.nih.gov/tsd/serials/lji.html
   Bibliographic information including standard abbreviations for serials
   indexed and cited in MEDLINE®

3 National Library of Medicine, United States
   http://www.nlm.nih.gov/pubs/factsheets/medline.html
   Provides access to MEDLINE® via PubMed®

4 PubMed Central
   http://www.pubmedcentral.nih.gov
   Provides access to archives of science journal literature

5 CrossRef
   http://crossref.org
   A collaborative reference linking service through which researchers can
   click on a reference citation in a journal and immediately access the cited
   article

6 Electronic Journal Miner
   http://ejournal.coalliance.org
   Website that allows you to search ejournals (both peer-reviewed and free
   publication)

7 Science Direct
   http://www.sciencedirect.com/
   Allows you to create a profile to search for references and receive alerts of
   new references as they become available

8 *Science Magazine*
   http://www.sciencemag.org/
   Provides access to the full text of *Science's* print version and to additional
   online-only enhancements; lets you search within *Science* and across a
   multitude of scientific journals; keeps you informed of new content and
   developments via email alerts, and helps you manage your citations

9 Institute for Scientific Information
   http://www.isiresearchsoft.com
   ISIResearchSoft provides product reviews and a comparison of the
   features of the three most widely used bibliographic software programs
   EndNote®, Reference Manager® and ProCite®

10 Medical College of Ohio, Raymon H. Mulford Library
    http://www.mco.edu/lib/instr/libinsta.html
    Links to websites that provide instructions to authors for over 2000
    journals in the health sciences

11 American Psychological Association
    http://www.apastyle.org/elecref.html
    http://www.apa.org/journals/1999_summary.html

Information of styles in which to cite references and information of the publication rates of many journals

12 Modern Language Association (MLA) of America
http://www.mla.org/
Guidelines for citing sources from the World Wide Web

13 *BMJ (British Medical Journal)*
http://www.bmj.com/advice/ index.html
Advice to authors and contributors on many issues of how to prepare papers for submission

14 *JAMA (Journal of the American Medical Association)* http://jama.ama-assn.org/issues/
Guidelines for writing papers reporting the results of diagnostic tests, cohort studies or case–control studies

15 Consolidated Standards of Reporting Trials
http://www.consort-statement.org/revisedstatement.htm
http://www.consort-statement.org/moose.pdf
http://www.consort-statement.org/quorom.pdf
Guidelines for reporting randomised controlled trials (CONSORT), Meta-analysis of Observational Studies in Epidemiology (MOOSE) and Quality of Reporting of Meta-analyses (QUORUM)

16 Cochrane Collaboration
http://www.cochrane.org/cochrane/hbook.htm
Guidelines for authors and contributors for preparing systematic reviews of the effects of healthcare interventions

References

1   Zeiger M. *Essentials of writing biomedical research papers*. Maidenhead: McGraw-Hill, 1991; p 9.
2   Rosner JL. Reflections of science as a product. *Nature* 1990;**345**:180.
3   Venter JC, Adams MD, Myers EW, *et al.* The sequence of the human genome. *Science* 2001;**292**:1304–51.
4   Lander ES, Linton LM, Birren B, *et al.* Initial sequencing and analysis of the human genome. *Nature* 2001;**409**:860–21.
5   David A. Write a classic paper. *BMJ* 1990;**300**:30–1.
6   Toelle BG, Peat JK, Salome CM, Mellis CM, Woolcock AJ. Toward a definition of asthma for epidemiology. *Am Rev Respir Dis* 1992;**146**: 633–7.
7   Peat JK, Haby MM, Spijker J, Woolcock AJ, Berry G. Busselton revisited. Abstract presented at Thoracic Society of Australia, Annual Scientific Meeting, Canberra, 1992.
8   Cunningham JD. Egotism in prestige ratings of Sydney suburbs: where I live is better than you think. *Aust J Psychology* 1984;**36**:429–38.
9   Institute of Clinical Evaluative Sciences. Twist and shout: deciding when to X-ray a sprained ankle. *Informed* 1994;**1**:1–2.
10 Siebers RW, Fitzharris P, Crane J. Beds, bedroom, bedding and bugs: anything new between the sheets? *Clin Exp Allergy* 1996;**26**:1225–7.
11 Tunstall-Pedoe H. Did MONICA really say that? *BMJ* 1998;**317**:1023.

12 Russell J, Baur L, Beument P, Byrnes S, Zipfel S. Refeeding of anorexics: wasteful not wilful. *Lancet* 1998;**352**:1445–6.
13 Forsen L, Meyer HE, Sogaard AJ, Naess S, Schei B, Edna TH. Mental distress and the risk of hip fracture. Do broken hearts lead to broken bones? *J Epidemiol Community Health* 1999;**53**:343–7.
14 Massel D. Similar, the same or just not different: a guide for deciding whether treatments are clinically equivalent. *Can J Cardiol* 1999;**15**: 556–62.
15 Greyson B. Dissociation in people who have near-death experiences: out of their bodies or out of their minds? *Lancet* 2000;**355**:460–2.
16 Mihrshahi S, Vukasin N, Forbes S, *et al.* for the CAPS team. Are you busy for the next 5 years? Recruitment in the Childhood Asthma Prevention Study. *Respirology* 2002;**7**:147–51.
17 Ke Y, Su B, Song X, *et al.* African origin of modern humans in East Asia: a tale of 12,000 Y chromosomes. *Science* 2001;**292**:1151–3.
18 Eckersley RM. Losing the battle of the bulge: causes and consequences of increasing obesity. *Med J Aust* 2001;**174**:590–2.
19 Cameron H, Robertson A. The colon in medicine: nothing to do with the intestinal tract. *BMJ* 1997;**315**:1657–8.
20 Rosner JL. Reflections of science as a product. *Nature* 1990;**345**:108.
21 Goodman NW. Survey of active verbs in the titles of clinical trial reports. *BMJ* 2000;**320**:914–15.
22 Smith R. Informative titles in the *BMJ*. *BMJ* 2000;**320**:915.
23 Weiss GB. New and improved titles. *J Clin Oncol* 1995;**13**:1829–30.
24 Lilleyman JS. Titles, abstracts, and authors. In: Hall GM. *How to Write a Paper, 2nd edition*. London: BMJ Publishing Group, 1994.
25 Siebers R, Holt S. Accuracy of references in five leading medical journals. *Lancet* 2000;**356**:1445.
26 Hall G. Structure of a scientific paper. In: *How to write a paper*. London: BMJ Publishing, 1997; pp 1–5.
27 Moher D, Schulz KF, Altman D, for the CONSORT group. The CONSORT statement: Revised recommendations for improving the quality of reports of parallel-group randomized trials. *JAMA* 2001;**285**:1987–91.
28 Toogood G. *The articulate executive*. Maidenhead: McGraw-Hill, 1995; p 113
29 Peat JK, Mellis CM, Williams K, Xuan W. Project management. In: *Health science research. A handbook of quantitative methods*. London: Allen and Unwin, 2001.

5: Review and editorial processes

If they have misunderstood your message, it is almost certainly your fault for not making things clear.

A David[1]

The objectives of this chapter are to understand how to:

- have insight into the editorial and external review processes
- follow the correct procedures to get your paper in print
- avoid problems with copyright and the press
- become a reviewer or an editor

Peer-reviewed journals

Peer review exists to keep egg off authors' faces.

S Goldbeck-Wood[2]

A peer-reviewed journal is one that is controlled by editorial staff who send papers out to external reviewers. The external reviewers are selected because they have a reputations as experts in their fields of research. The work that is published in peer-reviewed journals is considered far superior to that published in non-peer-reviewed journals simply because it has undergone expert external review. The editorial team has the responsibility of communicating with the author, and the external reviewers have the responsibility of ensuring that the external review process is rigorous and expeditious.

When you send your paper to a journal, there are usually two levels of review. The first is the internal peer review by the editorial team to decide whether your paper is the type of article that they want to see in their journal and, if so, whether it is of an adequate standard to be sent out for external review. Editors have the ultimate responsibility of selecting papers that will appeal to the journal's readership. At the *BMJ*, about half of the submitted papers are rejected in-house by the editorial committee[3] and at *JAMA* 42% of papers are rejected without external review.[4] Rejection is common and, perhaps for this reason, approximately half of the papers that are presented at conferences never make the grade to becoming a published journal article.[5]

Editors send papers out to external reviewers to ensure that only the strongest and most scientific work makes it through the net. Each paper is sent to only two or three reviewers but this may vary from journal to journal. The areas that reviewers are often asked to comment on are shown in Box 5.1. In addition, many journals ask reviewers to give a quality or priority ranking to various aspects of the paper. If the comments from two reviewers differ markedly, the editor will often ask for comments from an arbiter reviewer. The arbiter reviewer may be sent the prior review comments and asked to comment on both them and your paper.

Box 5.1 Reviewers are asked to comment on the following areas:

Scientific rigour
Experimental or study design
Adequacy of data
Importance and originality of the results
Validity of conclusions reached
Completeness of the literature cited
Clarity of writing
Interest to the journal readership

External reviewers are often asked to give useful advice to authors rather than make judgements on behalf of the editors. In this way, the integrity of the research, the quality of the journal and the development of the discipline are a combined responsibility of the editor, the reviewers, and the authors.[6] This process helps to shield busy researchers or clinicians from wasting their time reading inferior papers and helps to protect patients from the damaging effects of unreliable research.[2]

Once your paper is submitted to a journal, it becomes the property of the journal, and the editor has total discretion over who has access to it. Although letters from the editor to the reviewers often stress the confidential nature of papers under consideration, it is acceptable for external reviewers to pass papers on to colleagues for review. Thus, external reviewers are not always required to treat the papers sent to them with confidentiality. It is common practice for senior researchers to ask junior staff to review and comment on papers. In fact, editors often ask reviewers to do this if they do not have time to complete the external review themselves. However, to maintain standards, it is important that senior researchers supervise the review and approve the comments made.

Once the editorial committee receives the reviewers' comments, they classify the paper into one of several categories as shown in Box 5.2. Papers may be classified as unacceptable for publication on many grounds including poor science or reporting, inappropriate length, non-original results or material that is not appropriate for the journal. Editors are usually quite explicit in their correspondence about the reasons for their decisions.

Box 5.2 An editorial committee may decide that a paper:

Is acceptable for publication
Is acceptable for publication following minor revisions
Is acceptable for publication following major revision
May be reconsidered for publication following major revisions
May be considered for publication as a letter or a short report
Is unacceptable for publication

External review is designed to help editors select the best research for publication in their journals. As such, it is a confidential consultancy between the reviewer and the journal editor.[7] Although many authors think that they sometimes know who the reviewers are, this is often not the case. In a study of papers sent out to 252 external reviewers, less than 6% of the reviewers were correctly identified by authors.[8]

Until recently, the anonymity of reviewers was an integral part of the review process. This left reviewers free to make whatever criticisms they felt necessary. The editor then forwards the comments to the authors without the reviewers being directly accountable. This closed review system often comes under criticism, especially when authors feel that their manuscripts have been unfairly treated or even plagiarised.[9] Nevertheless, most authors and reviewers seem to be in favour of maintaining the reviewers' right to anonymity.[10]

To evaluate a more open peer-review system, the *BMJ* conducted a randomised controlled trial to test the effects of asking reviewers to consent to being identified to the authors. Interestingly, identification had no effect on the quality of the feedback received, on recommendations regarding publication, or on the time taken for the paper to be returned to the journal.[11] However, the thought of being identified significantly decreased the number of potential reviewers who consented to undertake a review. Despite the finding that this system was not detrimental to the quality of reviews, this type of open review is rarely conducted and anonymity is usually retained.

In an attempt to remove any bias due to lack of anonymity of authors to the reviewers, the *Medical Journal of Australia* conducted a trial of removing authors' names from papers sent out for external review. Once the paper was accepted for publication, the author and the reviewers were asked to consent to both the paper and the critical feedback being posted on the internet.[7] Selected email comments from readers were then added as commentary, and the authors could reply or revise their paper before it was finally published. An evaluation suggested that this open review system had some benefits such as increasing the fairness of the system and increasing the depth of feedback as a result of a wide range of readers posting their comments on the website. With the facilities that the internet offers, it seems likely that other journals may move to more open review methods in the future.

Revise and resubmit

> By the time I was fourteen (and shaving twice a week whether I needed to or not), the nail in my wall would no longer support the weight of the rejection slips impaled upon it. I replaced the nail with a spike and went on writing. By the time I was sixteen, I'd begun to get rejections slips with handwritten notes a little more encouraging.... (The first was from an editor who wrote) "This is good. Not for us, but good. You have talent. Submit again."
>
> Stephen King[12]

Once the review process is over, it is an exciting moment when you hear back from a journal. For some journals, you could hope to receive a letter with a preliminary decision within 3–4 months, but this process can often take much longer. Be patient, but not too patient. If you have not received a reply after 4 months, a polite letter to the editor enquiring about progress is in order. Many journals try to expedite the review process by getting consent from reviewers before dispatching the papers and by requesting faxed or email responses. However, the turnaround time can sometimes be slow and papers have occasionally gone missing.

It is very unusual to receive a letter that says that your paper has been accepted without some revisions being needed. You would probably have more chance of winning the lottery. The extent of the revisions requested can vary widely from minor additions to a radical shortening of the manuscript or inclusion of further analyses. Typical responses from an editor are shown in Box 5.3.

If the required revisions were extensive, the editor may send your revised paper back to the external reviewers for further comments after you have made the changes. The process then starts again and may again bring acceptance, further suggestions for change, or rejection. Many journals set a time limit of 3 or 6 months in which they are prepared to accept an amended version. If you resubmit after this time, your paper will in all likelihood be considered as an original submission.

Box 5.3 Typical letters of acceptance, or possible acceptance, from an editor

Your paper is now considered to be suitable for publication. You will receive the proofs in due course. You should correct these and return them to us as soon as possible. Once again, thank you for submitting your paper to our journal.

Thank you for submitting your paper to our journal. The reviewers to whom we sent your paper have made some important comments. If you are willing to address their comments adequately in a revised version of your paper, we should be happy to accept it for publication.

The editorial board has reviewed your manuscript. It is difficult to complete an editorial evaluation at this point in time. Major revisions are needed as noted in the enclosed comments. Please respond to each reviewer's comments point by point and resubmit your article to us.

Your manuscript has now been returned from our reviewers. As you can see from their enclosed comment, they have a number of suggestions, which they feel should be addressed before we are able to accept the manuscript for publication. If you are able to respond to these comments in an amended manuscript we shall then review the manuscript before final acceptance. Please let us know if you decide not to resubmit. If we have not heard from you in 3 months time, we will assume that you do not want to amend your manuscript and your file will be closed.

Three international reviewers have submitted comments about your manuscript. Together with the assistant chief editor, we generally agree with their remarks. If you would like to thoroughly revise the manuscript according to the combined suggestions, we should be happy to consider it again. Please submit the amended manuscript and three copies in addition to a copy of the original marked with the changes you have made within 3 months. Please appreciate that resubmission does not mean acceptance.

Remember that you can withdraw from a journal at any time but the withdrawal has to be formally accepted at editorial level before you can submit the paper to another journal. Deciding to withdraw and then submit to another journal will bring another set of reviewers' comments, albeit different ones, and will almost certainly delay the publication of your paper. If the paper is in a very specialised field, it may well find its way back to one of the original reviewers who will be less than impressed if you have not taken their original comments on board.

Replying to reviewers' comments

> *Education is what survives when what has been learnt has been forgotten.*

BF Skinner

When you receive the reviewers' comments, the extent of them may leave you feeling devastated. This is a normal response when unknown peers widely criticise many aspects of your work. The best approach is to be calm and objective. All you need to do is deconstruct each of the messages into individual items that you can respond to. In doing this, you will find that many comments are more easily responded to than at first thought. It is probably best to try and make the majority of the changes requested, and to try carefully to negotiate the more radical suggestions as needed. At the end of the line, editors take the review process very seriously so no comments from the reviewers should be lightly dismissed. Sending back a paper with minimal changes implies either disdain or arrogance for the review process and will not impress the journal editor.

Your replies to the reviewers' comments should make your responses very clear. This is the time to get the editorial panel on your side by simplifying the work they have to do in assessing your responses. Basically, you must take a positive attitude and put a lot of thought into your responses. A good way to respond is to use a table in which you list each of the reviewers' comments, your responses, and the amended text as shown in Table 5.1. This helps you to organise what you need to respond to. It also makes it very clear what you have done and why. It is a good idea to make most if not all of the changes suggested. You don't have to fully accept all suggestions but, if you don't, you need to give reasons that will convince the editor that your opinion is reasonable. In doing this, it is best to be pragmatic and not to be dismissive of the reviewers' work.

Tabulating the responses makes it very clear what changes you have made and where you have made them. In Table 5.1, most of the reviewers' comments have been accommodated. For comment 1, the reviewer's suggestion has been met half way by shortening the section considerably but still leaving some information in the paper. For comments 2, 5, 6, 8, and 9,

Table 5.1 Example of the use of a table to respond to reviewers' comments.

No.	Comment	Location	Amendment
1	The long section on avoidance of food allergens is not useful. The paragraphs should be deleted …	Page 3	This section has been shortened but not removed because one of the studies forms the basis of our hypothesis that diet modification may be important in reducing the incidence of asthma.
2	There should be discussion of the safety and possible side effects of Acaril	Page 5	A comment about the safety of Acaril has been added. Side effects of the active ingredient benzyl benzoate have only been reported when this compound has been applied directly to the skin or used to treat clothing at higher concentrations (10%). The concentration used in this study is 0·03% and is unlikely to cause these effects.
3	If sampling was by residential area, then there is a potential statistical issue to do with cluster designs	Page 6	We apologise for unintentionally being misleading. This study was not a cluster design and we have altered our wording accordingly. Children were selected who lived within a specified distance from the hospital. This has been made clear.
4	The method for calculating measurement error does not correspond to the coefficient of repeatability described by Bland and Altman in 1996	Page 7	We have calculated measurement error according to the method of Chinn (1991) and included the limits of agreement as described by Bland and Altman (1996).

(Continued)

Table 5.1 Continued

No.	Comment	Location	Amendment
5	The term "active group" may not be the best term	Throughout	The term has been changed to "intervention group" throughout.
6	Figure 2 is excellent but could be made clearer	Fig 2	We have made the suggested changes to Figure 2 and agree that this makes the figure easier to understand.
7	In my opinion, Figure 3 could be deleted	Fig 3	Figure 3 defines the allergen avoidance intervention in detail, as Figure 4 does the diet intervention. We have retained the figure but are happy for it to be deleted if the editor wishes to do this.
8	Setting the type I error rate at 0·05 does not avoid the possibility of a type I error, it just controls the error rate at not greater than 5%	Page 12	We have replaced the phrase "to avoid the possibility of a type II error" with "to control the type I error rate".
9	A summary paragraph would be helpful	Page 13	A summary paragraph has been added.

the reviewer's suggestions have been accommodated entirely. For comment 3, the response is to politely point out that the explanation of the sampling processes was unclear in the original paper and has been amended. In response to the reviewer's comment 4, it would be tempting to point out that Bland and Altman do not describe a "coefficient of repeatability" and that the reviewer might like to get his facts right! Nevertheless, you must always be polite. It is better to be certain that you have used the correct statistic and to just note what you have done, as in our reply. For comment 7, the decision has been left to the editor because the authors considered the figure to be essential to the message of the paper.

Occasionally, you find that the reviewer has made disparaging or less than polite comments. Remember that two wrongs do not make a right and that responding with disparaging or impolite comments will not impress the editor. It is best to be noble in the face of adversity. Occasionally reviewers may suggest that you include more work, seemingly forgetting that they are reviewing this paper and not the next one. This will take a prudent response, perhaps on advice from more senior researchers.

Handling rejection

As for disappointing them I should not so much mind; but I can't abide to disappoint myself.

Oliver Goldsmith (1728–1774)

Letters of rejection may arrive much more quickly than letters of acceptance because some journals may reject up to 50% of papers before they are sent out for external review. If your paper is rejected without being sent out for review, you could expect to hear back from the journal within a month. If your paper falls into this category, it is probably considered to be insufficiently original, to be of minor interest to the journal's readership, or to be scientifically flawed, too long, or incomprehensible. Editors strive to treat their external reviewers with respect and therefore do not send them papers that are perceived to be of poor quality.

Whether or not your paper has been sent out for external review, the letter you receive will be very polite if the editor decides to reject it. Some examples of rejection letters are shown in Box 5.4. If you receive this kind of letter, you need to swallow your pride. It happens to most writers at one time or another. Try to be optimistic and objective. You will need to decide whether the paper needs some major attention or whether you misjudged the appropriateness of the journal. Once a paper is formally rejected, you are free to submit it to another journal either without changes or with a complete rewrite.

Box 5.4 Typical letters of rejection from an editor

Thank you for sending us your revised manuscript. We have now considered this very carefully at an editorial level and I am afraid that we have decided not to accept the paper for publication. I know that you addressed the comments made by the reviewers by making some modifications to the paper. However, our decision not to publish was on the basis that we did not feel that the information was new or would be of great interest to our readership. I apologise for disappointing you.

Thank you for your communication that you sent for publication in our correspondence column. I am sorry to say that we will not be able to find room for it. With well over 2000 letters submitted every year, we sometimes have to make difficult editorial decisions.

Your manuscript has been reviewed. On the basis of the recommendations of the reviewers and the Editorial Office, it was not accepted. Both reviewers raised concerns regarding the study design, analysis, and interpretation of the data. We hope that you can use their comments to improve your manuscript for submission to another journal. Thank you for inviting us to consider your paper.

Thank you for resubmitting your manuscript. The further reports of the referees are enclosed and we hope that you will find them helpful. When evaluating whether a manuscript can be accepted for publication, the Editorial Office must consider several aspects such as scientific value, interest to readers, and space in the journal. Unfortunately, based on these factors and despite its scientific quality, your paper cannot be accepted for publication.

We have now received the reviewers' reports on your manuscript and enclose these for your information. We regret that we are unable to accept your paper in its present form. However, if you would like to revise your manuscript to address the reviewers' comments, we will resubmit it for review and will be happy to give it further consideration, although we cannot promise publication.

If the reviewers are critical of your basic methods, you may want to reconsider whether you can answer the question you set out to answer or whether the way you have presented the results is at variance with your aims. Solving these sorts of problems usually involves some serious rewriting and may involve further data analyses. If the comments relate to style and presentation, you would be wise to spend some time fixing these up before you reformat your paper for a new journal and resubmit it. However, after three consecutive rejections, it is perhaps prudent to completely reassess your whole approach.

Editorial process

> *"The editor is always right." The corollary is that no writer will take all of his or her editor's advice for all have sinned and fallen short of editorial perfection. Put another way, to write is human, to edit is divine.*
>
> Stephen King[12]

Once you have returned a revised paper to the journal, the editorial committee will consider the new version and your replies to the external reviewers' comments. At the *BMJ*, papers that are thought to merit publication at this stage are passed on to a very appropriately named "hanging committee". This committee is named after the committee at the Royal Academy in London that decides which pictures to hang in the summer exhibition each year. The hanging committee, which is made up of practising clinicians, statisticians, and medically qualified editors, makes the final decision about publication and may often ask for further revisions.

The entire editorial process is sometimes quite subjective. Editorial decisions may be made on many factors of which the external reviewers' comments are just one part. When a journal has a low publication rate, many papers have to be rejected. In the end, editors are likely to publish new, proactive, and interesting findings even if validity is in doubt, whereas papers that are more mundane have to have exceptional methods to even be considered. In addition, external reviewers may pass on confidential comments that contribute, rightly or wrongly, to editorial decisions and journals may lean heavily towards accepting papers that are likely to be cited regularly. It is a matter of bread and butter for the editors. Journals are often assessed by their impact factor (see Chapter 6). If the impact factor of the journal goes up then the quality and quantity of submissions also goes up, but if the impact factor goes down, then the good papers go elsewhere.

You may find that the reviewers' comments are not too damning, but that the editor has made his own decision to reject the paper anyway. Alternatively, the reviewers may have suggested fundamental changes to your paper, but the editor may be interested in publishing it. Publishing is essentially a competitive sport and journals often reject the majority of papers that they receive. The editor has absolute discretion over what is published. It pays to be philosophical and to be prepared to accept the vagaries of the editorial system.

The editorial process can sometimes be quite fluid and negotiable. If you think that you have an important new finding, you can ask the editor to expedite the review process or give you a rapid response on a publishing date. In this way, you may be able to fast track the publication of your results, although this doesn't happen often. If your paper is rejected or if you feel that the reviewers have overlooked or misunderstood something important, you can appeal against the editorial decision by writing a letter stating your case. It is rare that the decision will be overturned, but it has been known to happen. It is also possible for a paper to be formally accepted by a regional editor who sends you a letter of acceptance, and then be rejected at a later date by the editor-in-chief, although this very rarely happens.

Until the paper is published, nothing is certain. Most editors receive more papers than their journal could ever publish and take the pragmatic view that you will get your work published somewhere if it is good enough. If you do decide to appeal against a rejection decision, you will need to send a new copy of your paper to the editor because rejected papers do not remain on file.

Page proofs

Truth lies within a little and certain compass, but error is immense.

Viscount Bollingbrooke (1678–1751)

Page proofs, which are the typeset copy of your work, are exciting evidence of how your paper will look in the journal. Although it may take some months following acceptance of your paper for the page proofs, or galleys as they are sometimes called, to arrive, it is incredibly exciting to see tangible evidence of what your work will finally look like to the world. However, there is still more work to do. This is the time for the *final check*. Every word of every page needs to be read very slowly and very carefully to check for any typographical, printing or reporting errors. Because tables are often retyped before publishing, it is important to pay special attention to the formatting and content of your tables and figures because this is where most printing errors seem to occur. Errors in the paper when it appears in its published form will be entirely your responsibility.

During the printing process, a subeditor or copy editor may have reworded parts of your paper or rearranged your punctuation. Some journals remove all the commas, others add more in. You will have to live with this. When you receive the page proofs, your job is to ensure that all of the words and numbers are totally correct, but you cannot do more than make very simple changes. Although the temptation to just rewrite a bit here and add a bit there may be very strong, it is very unusual to be able to add more than a word or two at this stage. Attempts to make changes are entirely at the editor's discretion and, to discourage the practice, often incur substantial page charges. Some journals also charge manuscript processing fees or page fees either for the entire paper or for a number of pages above a specified threshold.

The journal will send you specific proof reading instructions that must be followed. Page proofs usually need to be marked with standard proofreading marks. If you are unsure of which marks to use or what each mark means, a copy of proof marks can be purchased online from the British Standards Institute (BSI) (www[1]). The BSI proofreading marks, which were first published in 1976, have become a widely accepted standard for the preparation and correction of documents. A number of websites also provide information or variations on the standard proofreading marks (www[2-5]).

Copyright laws

*There are some things about which we must simply say
you can't do.*

James Watson (codiscoverer of DNA, b. 1928)

Copyright is a law that protects writers from having their
work copied without permission. Any person who copies
protected material without the copyright owner's
permission is infringing the copyright laws. International
conventions on copyright have been incorporated into
domestic law to establish who owns the copyright of a
research article. In part, this law was devised to ensure that
the writer of a piece of work is always justly attributed as
being the writer. However, the copyright laws have some
practical aspects. If you are a researcher, you are allowed to
copy any copyright material for the purpose of your
research, and you do not infringe copyright if your use is
fair. In general, your institution will own the copyright of
draft papers that are being written to publish research
conducted in the institution, but this copyright is
automatically assigned to a journal once you have submitted
your paper there.

A paper is under strict copyright restrictions from the time
that it is first submitted to a journal. Thus, you need to be
very careful about giving copies of your manuscript to
researchers who are not coauthors. A slogan across the front
that says *This article is confidential and is under strict copyright
restrictions – do not copy under any circumstances* should get the
message across.

Once the paper is published, some journals allow you to put
copies of your paper on your personal website, but not until
3 years after publication. However, you are not allowed to scan
in the final published copy or download the final electronic
copy. Also, you may post your paper on your personal website
but must not post it on a department, university, or corporate
website. If you are unsure of the copyright restrictions of your
journal, always contact them for clarification.

Releasing results to the press

"All the news that's fit to print." Motto of the New York Times.

Adolph Ochs (1858–1935)

You should never release your research results to the press before they appear in print in the journal. Journals do not want to publish work that has already appeared in detail in the mass media. Although there can be a long period between presenting an abstract at a conference and the appearance of a paper in a journal, you should not be tempted to participate in press conferences or issue a press release about your findings prior to publication. Indeed, some journals will not take papers that have been disseminated as full reports in conference proceedings, and a paper may be rejected outright or withdrawn from publication if it is given media coverage before it is published.

As an author, you may have presented your work widely at meetings, published abstracts, and attended press conferences to discuss your results. It is generally agreed that press communications in the context of a scientific conference are an important part of the scientific process but that they are not publications in the proper sense. Researchers should feel free to discuss their presentations with the media but should not offer more detail than they included in the presentation. Fortunately, press reports are not usually regarded as breaches, as long as they do not contravene embargo regulations and as long as they are fairly general and do not include exact replicas of the tables or figures that you submit in your paper. It pays to be very conservative about where you publicise any early results.

Despite the fact that the press often reports new findings from scientific meetings, any research results should be considered preliminary until the full report of the study undergoes peer review and is considered worthy of publication. For this reason, some journals have strict policies regarding prepublication of research results to overcome the conflict between the news media, who strive to publish any new information as quickly as possible, and the journal editors, who prefer to disseminate research information only after validation by peer review. Although journals have been criticised for exerting too much control over the release of research results to the media, they go to great lengths to ensure the accuracy and validity of the information they publish.[13]

The Ingelfinger rule

Releasing data to the media prior to publication will violate the copyright policy of most journals. This policy, which is commonly known as the "Ingelfinger rule", dates back to the 1960s. Franz Ingelfinger, who was the editor of the *New England Journal of Medicine* at that time, objected to papers being reported in the free press before they were published in the subscription based journal.[14] Although the Ingelfinger rule was introduced to protect the newsworthiness of journals, it is now used to defend the value of peer review in assessing the scientific validity of research findings.

The Ingelfinger rule, which covers embargoes on prepublication, has been adopted by many journals despite ongoing controversy about its influence on delaying the release of important research results to the public. In response, researchers may decide to withhold their full results at conferences where information is available to the media to ensure that their work is publishable.[15]

Embargoes

The embargo is a time during which the authors agree to not discuss their findings with the press before their paper is published and distributed. Many journals will place an embargo on your paper prior to publication and will include details of their embargo in your contract. In practice, an embargo limits prepublication publicity and protects both the authors and the publishers. In essence, the embargo allows you to prepare for the impact of the release of your results to the public and thus to avoid misinterpretation. It is in everyone's interest to respect embargoes. When embargoes are broken, people who have a vested interest in the study results are not able to obtain the information that they expect and the researchers who plan to disseminate results in a careful and responsible manner are undermined.[16]

An embargo means that a preliminary release of your data may take place only with consent from the editor and will be granted only in situations such as a public health emergency.[17] Traditionally, a scientific paper has been deemed to be published once it appears in a paper journal and publication is defined as the moment that the embargo is lifted. Most journals have specific times when their embargo is lifted. For example the *BMJ* lifts its embargo at 00·01 hours on Fridays and the *JAMA* typically holds its embargoes until 15·00 hours on the day before the cover date of the journal.[18]

To satisfy embargoes about releasing data to the press and fulfilling journal requirements, some researchers go to extraordinary lengths to work together with journal editors to publish their results at the same time that the results are presented at a conference and released on a website.[19] It is a good idea to be wary of the problems of prepublication and press releases, and always to check with your journal before you release any information to the media or onto the web.

Becoming a reviewer

Serving as a reviewer or editor allows you to shape your field – publishing good work and keeping bad science out of the literature.

McCabe and McCabe[20]

Once you have started publishing, it is fun to start reviewing. Although this honorary position rarely brings financial rewards, it is exciting to be invited to be an external reviewer by a journal. In fact, if you write, then you should also be willing to review. However, reviewing is a serious undertaking and can be time-consuming when done properly. In being a good reviewer, you need time to read the paper carefully from beginning to end, think about it, read it a second time, write a review, revise your review, and then check back with the paper again. The rewards for this are that you are sent the most current research work to read and that your reviewing skills have a currency that help to foster good science in the journals as well as your career.

Many journals hold large databases of reviewers, most of whom will be sent a review only once or twice each year.[4] Many journals, but not all, will contact you to ask whether you can undertake the review before they send the paper to you. You should only accept papers for review if you have no conflict of interest and if you can complete the review within the suggested time frame, which can be as little as 2 weeks. It is important that you do not unduly delay manuscripts. Typical letters that you may receive from an editor are shown in Box 5.5.

Box 5.5 Typical letters from editors to reviewers

I know you must be frightfully busy, but I have received the enclosed manuscript and I think you could give a balanced and reasonable review of this work. I would be very grateful to receive your confidential comments about the suitability of this work for inclusion in our journal. I enclose two sets of referee sheets, one of which will be sent to the authors and the other retained by the journal. I would appreciate it if I could receive your comments within the next 3 weeks.

Thank you for agreeing to review the above article. Please complete the enclosed referee checklist (it is a guide only, not all aspects will be applicable to all manuscripts) and provide detailed comments based on the referee checklist that will help us to make a decision about the article. These comments may be sent to authors in order to help them revise the manuscript. We should appreciate receiving your review by email or fax in the next 2 weeks. Thank you very much for undertaking this work for our journal; it is very much appreciated.

Thank you very much for reviewing the above manuscript. The authors have revised the manuscript along with our joint comments. I would greatly value your reassessment of the manuscript with a focus on the adequacy of the response to the points that you raised earlier. Please find enclosed the marked-up version of the new document and the responses to the reviewers' comments.

We are very grateful for your thoughtful and detailed review and comments on the paper that we recently sent to you. On reflection and after discussion with the authors, they have made changes but not as extensive as you suggested. The paper is one of a series and, at an editorial level, we believe that the general style is appropriate for our journal. Thank you for your review but, as you will understand, we have elected to proceed with publication with some of your suggestions incorporated.

To expedite the review process, most journals now accept reviews by email or fax. If you do not complete the review within the allocated time period, you will more than likely receive a prompt reminder. Some journals have a "screening review for rapid rejection" that reviewers can use to reject manuscripts within 3 days if the paper is clearly not suitable for consideration for publication. Once your review is completed, the manuscript should be returned to the journal or destroyed depending on journal policy. If a journal asks the authors to make substantial changes to their paper in response to your comments, you may receive the paper for a second round of reviewing after it has been amended. At this time, you will be required to consider the authors' responses to your comments and to perform a new review of the paper. This process may take more time than the original review but is essential in the review process.

If you are too busy to undertake a review, you may choose to pass the manuscript on to a more junior staff member for comment, as is allowed and often suggested by editors. Before the review is returned, it is important that you approve the comments made. You must also acknowledge this contribution when returning the manuscript to the editor. In this way, the junior researcher receives the credit deserved, and this, in turn, can help to ease them gently into the system and to foster their reputation.

As a reviewer, you can contact the editor at any time to request information about the progress of a paper. Once a decision has been made about publication, many journals send a copy of the reply to the authors and copies of all reviewers' comments to each reviewer. Some journals may ask you to write an editorial, leading paper, or comment for the same edition in which the paper will appear. This brings a bonus of an immediate and ensured publication on a current hot topic.

Writing review comments

As an editor, David [David Sharp, former editor of Lancet] worked on all sections of the Lancet. *He believed in plain language ... As a teacher, he had exacting standards. Many an overconfident doctor arrived at the* Lancet *sure that aptitude with a scalpel rendered the pen a trivial challenge, only to be shown the true meaning of humility.*

Richard Horton[21]

Being a good reviewer is something that experts, or experts in training, are automatically expected to know how to do. Once you have established your research reputation, you will be asked to review papers that fall within your own area of expertise. The journal editor may give you some ideas of what to be on the look out for, will ask you to rank the quality of the paper in various ways, or may even send you a checklist. A list of commonly used checklist questions was shown in Box 4.5.

As a reviewer, your job is to assess the scientific merit of the paper. You may be asked to rank your feedback under general comments, or under comments that recommend major or minor revisions. You must ensure that your comments are listed on the comment summary sheets and your ratings on the rating summary sheets. Writing comments on the pages of the paper is not useful since most editors will not want to inspect every page of every copy that they send out for review[22] and they do not send marked-up copies back to the authors.

As a reviewer, you can make general comments about style but do not need to address specific problems with punctuation, grammar, spelling, etc. These problems will be addressed by the editor in deciding whether to accept the paper and by the copy editors when typesetting the paper. It is important that external reviewers treat these issues sensitively especially for authors who are from a non-English speaking background. Nevertheless, you will need to take a general overview of the presentation, the spelling, and the grammar, since this will give you some insight as to whether the writer has paid attention to detail and whether the paper can be made interesting and readable if the writing is improved. Lack of attention to detail is not a good quality in scientific research.

Most of your review comments should deal with the more substantive issues of content, science, and interpretation. If you are unsure whether the statistics are sound, you can ask the editor to call a biostatistician into the process. In writing your review, be polite and constructive at all times. Although your review will be anonymous, you should write as though you were being made known to the authors. Remember also that most editors maintain databases of the style, reliability, and judgements of their reviewers. If you want a respected position on the database, you will need to write critical responses that are polite, considered, and helpful to both the editor and the authors.

Some examples of the types of comments made by reviewers are shown in Box 5.6. In all review comments, it helps to state the problem as you perceive it and a possible solution. It also helps to number your comments so that the authors can make it clear how they have responded to each of them. Finally, you may have the option of giving a short opinion to the editors that is not passed on to the authors. This is the place where you can make cryptic comments about the quality of the paper that would be too blunt to send to the authors. Comments such as *I cannot see what relevance these data would have to clinical care*, or *This article is long, lacks focus and is badly planned and written* are fine to send to the editor. On the other hand, comments such as *This paper reports exciting results and with a few amendments will make an excellent journal article* are welcomed by both editors and authors. Whatever happens, your comments to the editor and the authors should not be at variance with one another in judging the publishable status of the paper. Good reviewers do not send positive messages to authors and leave the editor to break the bad news that the paper is not going to be published.

It is a good feeling when authors make the changes requested and reviewers can write feedback such as *The revisions that the authors have made have improved this paper considerably. The analyses are logical for answering the study aims, the limitations of the study are discussed, and the conclusions are a reasonable interpretation of the results presented.* This is confirmation that writing and reviewing are complementary processes that promote the publication of high quality scientific papers.

Box 5.6 Examples of reviewer's comments

The response rate for the study is not given. This needs to be included and the authors need to present some data to verify the representativeness of their sample. A sensitivity analysis to allow the reader to gauge the effects of selection bias on the prevalence rates reported would be helpful.

Many subgroup analyses are presented, although the small numbers in some groups and the wide confidence intervals indicate a lack of statistical power to test the relationships. The subgroup analyses should preferably be deleted or the authors need to discuss the extent to which the results presented could be type II errors.

The tables are long and present far too much data to be readily understood. Many outcome variables are presented, which must overlap to a great extent in individuals. The data would be better summarised into exclusive groups that are categorised according to the multiplicity or severity of symptoms. This would give readers a much clearer idea of the burden of illness in the population studied.

The analyses have been stratified by gender although there is no *a priori* reason to suggest a gender difference and the rates of illness appear similar between the genders. Gender effects would be better tested in a single model unstratified analysis, and this would have the additional benefit of improving precision around the estimates of effect.

I can find no evidence in the results to support the conclusion that adenoidectomy may influence immune development. This conclusion seems to be speculative and therefore should be removed.

Becoming an editor

> *When I asked him [David Sharp, former* Lancet *editor] what he had enjoyed most during his* Lancet *years, he replied "The craft of editing" ... David's love, for it was that, of our craft inspired colleagues over several decades.*
>
> Richard Horton[21]

Editors are appointed by the journal's financial owners. The journal's owners, who are responsible for making business decisions, may be concerned about many performance indicators of their journal such as circulation rates, advertisements placed, negative and positive feedback from readers, the number of papers submitted, the number of mentions in the press, and so on. Journals naturally select editors who can maintain or improve these indicators. Because editorial independence is valued highly by both readers and subscribers, the hiring and firing of editors is sometimes debated publicly because it raises questions about editorial freedom, the cultures of journals, and the relationship between a journal and its owners.[23]

Being an editor at the helm of the review process is a heady occupation. Editors have full authority for determining the content of the journal and for pleasing the target readership. Readers not only want short articles that are easy to read but they must feel confident that the articles are accurate, informative, and up to date. It is the job of the editor to entice potential readers of the journal to pick it up, open it, start reading, keep reading, and, even better, look forward to the next issue.[22]

An editor is responsible for making critical decisions about publication of papers and correspondence. It is the editor's responsibility to select reviewers carefully, to ensure that their comments are polite and constructive, to rank areas of priority for publication, and to answer specific questions from authors. Following feedback from reviewers and responses from the authors, the editor has the task of trying to balance the two sources of comments, and adjudicate the final decision about publication. This is sometimes difficult when two of the external reviewers have opposing opinions and, ultimately, the editor has to take responsibility for accepting or disregarding reviewers' comments. When decisions become especially difficult, the editor may refer the paper to an independent advisory committee who considers issues that are contentious or perceived as malpractice.

It takes a long time for journals to establish their reputations and to increase their impact factors and it is the editor's job to maintain or improve these. An editor is sometimes selected on the basis of the reviews that they have undertaken for a journal. Some journals require that potential editors have performed a certain number of reviews each year to establish commitment before they can become involved in the editorial process. Other journals select editors on the basis of their reputation or through an election process. If you want to become an editor, it is probably best to ask a senior colleague for advice about how to get there.

Acknowledgements

King quotes have been reprinted with the permission of Scribner, a Division of Simon & Schuster, Inc., from *On Writing: A Memoir of the Craft* by Stephen King. Copyright © by Stephen King. The Skinner Goldsmith, Bollingbrooke, Watson and Ochs quotes have been produced with permission from *Collins Concise Dictionary of Quotations* 3*rd* edn. London: Harper Collins, 1998 (p 299, 174, 54, 159, 228 respectively). All other referenced quotes have been produced with permission.

Websites

1 *British Standards Institute (BSI)*
   http://www.bsi-global.com/index.html
   Standard proofreading marks for the copy preparation and proof correction of documents. Standard number: BS 5261C: 1976

2 *Capital Community College, Hartford, CO, USA*
   http://webster.commnet.edu/writing/symbols.htm
   Provides a table of common proofreading symbols

3 *Accurate Design & Communications, Ottawa, Canada*
   http://www.accurate.on.ca/html/features/proofread.html
   Provides a table of proofreading symbols with descriptions and examples

4 *Boston College, Chestnut Hill, MA, USA*
   http://www.bc.edu/bc_org/omc/resources_marks.html
   Provides a list of proofreading symbols with descriptions and examples

5 *University of Oregon, USA*
   http://uopress.uoregon.edu/tools/proofmarks.shtml
   Contains a list of proofreading marks that are used to indicate corrections and changes to proof pages. An Adobe Acrobat version of these proofreading marks can be downloaded

References

1 David A. Write a classic paper *BMJ* 1990;**300**:30–1.
2 Goldbeck-Wood S. What makes a good reviewer of manuscripts? *BMJ* 1998;**316**:86.
3 Editorial. Getting published in the BMJ: advice to authors. *BMJ* 1997;**314**:66–8.
4 Williams ES. The *JAMA* peer review report for 2000. *JAMA* 2001;**285**:1078.

5   Petticrew M, Gilbody S, Song F. Lost information? The fate of papers presented at the 40th Society for Social Medicine Conference. *J Epidemiol Community Health* 1999;**53**:442–3.
6   Morse JM. "Revise and resubmit": responding to reviewers' reports. *Qual Health Res* 1996;**6**:149–51.
7   Bingham CM, Higgins G, Coleman R, van der Weyden MB. The Medical Journal of Australia internet peer-review study. *Lancet* 1998;**352**:441–5.
8   Wessely S, Brugha T, Cowen T, Smith L, Paykel E. Do authors know who refereed their paper? A questionnaire survey. *BMJ* 1996;**313**:1185.
9   Rennie D. Freedom and responsibility in medical publication. Setting the balance right. *JAMA* 1998;**280**:300–2.
10 Hearse DJ. Anonymity of reviewers – editorial comment. *Cardiovas Res* 1994;**28**:1133.
11 van Rooyen S, Godlee F, Evans S, Black N, Smith R. Effect of open peer review on quality of reviews and on reviewers' recommendations: a randomised trial. *BMJ* 1999;**318**:23–7.
12 King S. *On writing.* London: Scribner, 2000; pp 41, 134.
13 Fontanarosa PB, Flanagin A. Pre-publication release of medical research. *JAMA* 2000;**284**:2927–9.
14 Altman LK. The Ingelfinger rule, embargoes, and journal peer review – part 1. *Lancet* 1996;**347**:1382–6.
15 Rosenberg SA. Secrecy in medical research. *N Engl J Med* 1996;**334**:392–4.
16 Peschanski M. The breaking of embargoes. *Lancet* 2001;**357**:963.
17 International Committee of Medical Journal Editors. Uniform requirements for manuscripts submitted to biomedical journals. *Ann Intern Med* 1997;**126**:36–47.
18 Fontanarosa PB, Flanagin A, DeAngelis CD. The journal's policy regarding release of information to the public. *JAMA* 2000;**284**:2929–31.
19 Holman R. Authors' choice of study was ill informed. *BMJ* 2001;**321**:1078.
20 McCabe, McCabe. *How to succeed in academics.* New York: Academic Press, 2000; p 127.
21 Horton R. The *Lancet* – now less Sharp. *Lancet* 2001;**357**:1820.
22 Ellard J. How to make an editor's life easier. *Australasian Psychiatry* 2001;**9**:212–14.
23 Rennie D. Editors and owners – stretching reputation too far. *JAMA* 1999;**282**:783–4.

6: Publishing

Writing for a readership imposes certain disciplines on the writer, such as the need to be intelligible and interesting, the need to order your material in a cogent and consistent way, and the need for clarity of expression in your choice of words and phrases. With practice, this discipline helps you learn how to craft your writing to suit your target audience.

Irina Dunn[1]

The objectives of this chapter are to understand how to:

- avoid duplicate publication
- share data in large research teams
- use the electronic media appropriately
- assess the merit of journals and journal articles

Duplicate publication

A scientific paper is (1) the first publication of original research results, (2) in a form whereby peers of the author can repeat the experiments and test the conclusions, and (3) in a journal or other source document readily available with the scientific community.

Infection and Immunity[2]

Redundant or duplicate publication occurs when results that are published in one paper substantially overlap with results published in another. This must be avoided at all costs. Duplicate publication is unnecessary and is usually fraudulent since the authors have given a signed assurance that their work has not been published elsewhere. If you have any related information that is published in or has been submitted to another journal then you should include it when you submit your paper. In this way, it becomes the editor's responsibility if the journal accepts a piece of work that proves to be duplicated. If more than 10% of a paper overlaps with another paper, the International Committee of Medical Journal Editors[3] asks you to send in copies of the other paper so that the editorial panel can make an informed decision about the extent of any duplication of published data.

No journal wants to publish papers that duplicate data that are already in press in another journal. If you want to include previous data analyses in your paper, the correct process is to cite them in the reference list. In some cases, secondary publication in another language is justifiable but only with the permission of the journal editor who may impose certain conditions. Most journals specifically ask authors to declare that their data are not published elsewhere and are not under consideration by another journal. These declarations help to prevent violation of copyright laws and to protect readers from being overwhelmed with information that is already in press.

It is especially important not to present closely related analyses from the same study to two journals concurrently without disclosure to both journal editors.[4] Closely related analyses sometimes go unnoticed in the literature and may be published with the intent of reaching different audiences. However, duplicate publication that comes to the notice of an editor will result in a prompt rejection and may result in disciplinary action from your institution or professional body. If the data are already in press, then a notice of duplicate publication may be published in the journal, perhaps without you as the author being given any prior notice. Such notices may also indicate withdrawal of the publication from the journal,[5] which means that the article will be tracked by indexing services such as MEDLINE® as withdrawn. Most importantly, some editors have a strict policy of rejecting all future publications from authors who have submitted duplicate data to their journal.

Most journals readily give permission for the reproduction of published figures and tables for which they have copyright, provided that the work is formally cited. However, you should be very careful when submitting data that are published in conference proceedings or in similar formats.

Some journals will not regard this as duplicate publication but others may be more restrictive. However, the rules of duplicate publication do not preclude you from submitting a paper that contains data presented as an abstract or oral communication at a scientific meeting or a paper that has been rejected by another journal. It is generally accepted that results presented at scientific meetings in order to elicit peer review are from preliminary analyses and are not published in full. Scientific meetings are organised in order that researchers can exchange information with one other and are not primarily intended as a venue for releasing results to the public.[6]

Reporting results from large studies

> I have read that more than 100,000 medical journals are being published currently … Whole libraries of medical books are published each year … On top of all that is information from the Royal Colleges, the AMA, the medical defence organisations and a dozen or so other worthy bodies … There is endless material from the pharmaceutical companies and then there is the Net. Doctors are not deprived of information, they are drowning in it.
>
> John Ellard[7]

In many studies, especially large epidemiological or multicentre studies, the publication of more than one paper from a study is often justified. Publication may begin with a paper about a new method that was developed for the purpose of the study. This can then be followed by papers in which results directly related to the study aims are reported, perhaps in sequential stages. Further papers may follow that fulfil aims that were not planned when the study began but for which the data are appropriate. Although practices such as testing for all relationships between all variables (so called "data-dredging") are unscientific, it is acceptable to make economical use of data that have been expensive to collect and that are appropriate for answering new questions.

Box 6.1 shows the first three publications from a large epidemiological study conducted in two countries. The first paper reported the development of a new questionnaire to measure the prevalence of chronic, persistent cough in epidemiological studies of children. The second and third papers report data from studies in which the questionnaire was used. The second paper was used to report evidence that children with symptoms of persistent cough do not have the same clinical features as children with clinically recognised asthma. Finally, in the third paper, the prevalence and risk factors for asthma and allergic illness in the two different countries was compared. Each paper has a clear, individual message and avoids the duplicate publication of data in the other papers. This process makes sense because the results reported in the three papers answer discrete questions and could not have been compressed into the constraints of a single paper. Because it was unlikely that one journal would have taken all three papers, each journal was chosen because the paper fell within its scope.

Box 6.1 Example of justified publications from a large, epidemiological study

1 Faniran AO, *et al*. Measuring persistent cough in epidemiological studies: development of a questionnaire and assessment of prevalence in two countries. *Chest* 1999;**115**:434–9.
2 Faniran AO, *et al*. Persistent cough – is it asthma? *Arch Dis Child* 1998;**79**:411–14.
3 Faniran AO, *et al*. Prevalence of atopy, asthma symptoms and diagnosis, and the management of asthma: comparison of an affluent and a non-affluent country. *Thorax* 1999;**54**:606–10.

Policies for data sharing

Premature release of research data before careful analysis of results, and without the independent scientific peer review that is part of the normal process of publication of scientific research, would also increase the risk of public disclosure of erroneous or misleading conclusions and confuse the public.

Bruce Alberts (President of the National Academy of Sciences, www.nationalacad-emies.org)

Data sharing often occurs in large studies when the data are used by more than one researcher to answer different questions. In many large research studies from which more than one paper will be published, strict policies are needed for data sharing to avoid duplicate publication and to specify each researcher's rights and responsibilities. It is the duty of the stakeholders in these studies to make collective decisions, in advance, about many aspects of publication. The stakeholders will include the principal investigators and other researchers, such as the divisional or departmental head, the project coordinator, the data manager, the research assistants, research fellows, postdoctoral students, and/or a statistician, etc. The decisions will include which questions will be answered, which dependent and independent variables will be used, which journals to select for publication, which national or international meetings the data will be presented at, and who will write the paper and present the data.

One good way to handle data sharing is to create a log sheet for each proposed paper. Box 6.2 shows some examples of the sort of information that can be included in publication log sheets. The log sheets should be formal documents that are agreed to by all stakeholders and that are formally archived in the study handbook.[8] Any changes to the log sheets must be approved at management meetings of the stakeholders and should be noted in the minutes of the meeting. Once the questions to be answered in the paper are finalised and the log sheet has been approved by the stakeholders, data sharing becomes plain sailing. In a perfect world, data sharing log sheets would be used routinely in all research studies.

Box 6.2 Suggested content of data sharing log sheets

Title of proposed paper
Author list
Specific research questions
Outcome and explanatory variables to be used in analyses
Details of data analyses and statistical methods
Details of database and file storage names
Journals chosen for submission
Acknowledgements of individuals, funding bodies, statistical advice, etc.
Conferences where data will be presented and by whom

This level of organisation often makes the difference between an everyday research team and a highly successful research team.

As discussed in Chapter 2, the first author must take full responsibility for preparing the paper. This author will be responsible for supervising or conducting the data analyses, documenting the results, and preparing the drafts of the paper, abstracts, posters, etc. The first author should also have the first option of presenting the results at scientific meetings. However, all stakeholders should have access to results for use in reviews, talks, research reports, etc. provided that this does not jeopardise the presentation or publication rights of the first author. When data are used by other stakeholders in this way, the first author should be acknowledged accordingly.

Data sharing has the potential to cause many emotional and professional conflicts. For this reason, academic departments and research teams need to work collaboratively to form their own data sharing policies in a consensus forum. It is crucial that a consensus is reached at the outset of the study. Such policies need to be approved by the divisional or departmental head and/or other people who have the responsibility of administering research policies and mediating any problems that occur. Only the adoption of a sensible and collaborative management approach can ensure that the issues of intellectual property, data sharing, and authorship are handled in a way that is rewarding for all of the parties involved.

Fast tracking and early releases

> In science read, by preference, the newest works; in literature, the oldest.
>
> Edward Bulwer-Lytton (1803–1873)

If you think that your results are exciting and important and that they need to be published quickly, it is sometimes possible to queue-jump and expedite publication. If you feel that your work needs to be published quickly, you can contact the editors of your journal of choice and put this thought to them, or consider writing a rapid communication. If you ask the editor to fast track your paper, you can expect one of three possible answers that will arrive back to you within days. The possible answers are outright rejection of your paper, a fast track review, or a standard external review. If your paper is accepted as a rapid communication, it will be dealt with swiftly by the editorial committee and, once accepted, may well appear in the next issue of the journal that is published.

Rapid communications are generally much shorter than standard journal articles and are used to report original work that is of immediate importance to the scientific community. However, rapid communications are stand-alone articles that should not be used to make a preliminary report of new work that you want to publish in more detail at a later date. A rapid communication can be cited in a future paper but the work cannot be repeated in more detail in a subsequent original journal article because this would be considered to be duplicate publication.

Some journals, such as the *New England Journal of Medicine*, have a policy of releasing some papers early by posting them on their website.[9] Such papers are released approximately two months earlier than the printed journal. In this process, the electronic and printed versions of the papers are identical. The decision to release a paper early is made together with the authors and is usually adopted only for papers that may have immediate implications for clinical practice.

Electronic journals and e-letters

The revolution in biomedical publishing is just a mouse click away.

Rebecca Voelker[10]

Many journals, including the *BMJ* and the *New England Journal of Medicine*, now publish papers in electronic form on the world wide web as well as in paper copy.[11] One advantage of electronic publishing is that it makes journal articles quickly and widely available throughout the world, which cannot be achieved in printed form.

In an attempt to please both medical practitioners who like short articles and researchers who like more detail, the *BMJ* sometimes publishes shorter versions of articles in its paper journal and longer versions in the electronic journal (*eBMJ*). These two publication modes cater to very different audiences.[11] However, it can be confusing when readers access only the shorter, printed version that may not include essential details. For example, the paper version of a study omitted the details of how the results were adjusted for the cluster method of randomisation, although this was included in the electronic version.[12] This elicited three critical letters that were posted on the web within 24 hours of receipt by the journal. The principal authors then had to respond quickly to each communication to avoid the paper being dismissed on unfair grounds by readers of e-letters. If the journal in which you publish has a rapid response feature, you may need to set some time aside following publication to deal with any immediate electronic correspondence.

Rapid response features mean that most electronic responses are posted on the web in a very short time period, often within seven days. This substantially increases the amount of feedback to authors because most of the correspondence relating to both electronic and paper articles is posted on the web compared with only 15% of correspondence that is eventually published in the paper journal. Although replying to correspondence is time consuming, good science relies on peer review. Also, interactive feedback avoids delays of up to six months that sometimes occurs before letters are published in a printed journal.[13]

Electronic post-publication review, which makes every reader a potential reviewer, is a level of peer review that was not previously available.[14] Post-publication review in an interactive environment in which authors can make changes in response to criticisms from readers will require increased accountability from authors. In response to the benefits that electronic review can offer, the *Medical Journal of Australia* has been placing some articles on the web, while they are still under editorial review. This allows for pre-publication review from the readership and subsequent revision by authors before papers are accepted and published. It will be interesting to see how journals change in the next few years in response to the interactive pre- and post-publication review facilities that the web offers.

Online journals have the advantage that they give researchers and clinicians more immediate access to the latest research information.[10] Electronic journals also cost less to produce, although the cost saving may not be passed on to the subscribers. Electronic publishing can be especially useful to some groups, such as researchers and health professionals who have delayed access to paper journals, who work in countries where paper journals are not freely available, or who have access to the web but are unable to attend conferences.

The Public Library of Science has set up a series of electronic journals that will publish peer-reviewed articles that will be freely accessible from the moment of publication (www[1]). With the advent of electronic publishing, some research groups have begun to challenge the ownership of papers by journals. Journals such as *Nature* and *Science* take the problem seriously and have e-debates about this on their websites (www[2,3]). An advocacy group of researchers is urging scientific publishers to pass research articles from their journals on to public online archives within six months of publication (www[4]). This move is supported by thousands of scientists but is not supported by the journals who argue that they cannot protect journal articles from misuse unless they own the copyright. It will be interesting to see where the debate leads.

With the advent of electronic publishing, journals are being forced to rethink their business models and plan for lower subscriptions as readers and libraries move to electronic access. Instead of billing readers, some journals are considering billing authors in the form of page charges. Although the move to electronic publishing is progressing rapidly, many researchers do not appreciate the extra time that it takes to monitor, search, and acquire electronic information and many groups remain convinced that paper journals are here to stay.

Netprints

We think of publishers as being like a midwife. They are paid for their role and, at the end of the day, they give the baby back to the parents.

Michael Eisen (Public Library of Science initiator, www[1])

Netprints, or e-prints, are electronic articles that are available in online journals. An advantage of netprints is that the results of a study become available to researchers much more quickly than through the standard journal process of review and publication.[15] This is also a disadvantage when the articles do pass through an external peer-review process. At some sites, authors are able to post their work before, during, or after review by other agencies (www[5,6]). The publication of netprints, which allows researchers to share their results as soon as their study is complete, is acceptable to many journals. In some cases, netprints may graduate to publication in standard journals when they are not considered to infringe copyright. The response to netprint sites has not been as vigorous as at first hoped and there is no suggestion at the moment that netprints will replace the role of peer-reviewed journals.

It has been argued that netprints are not very different from presenting a paper at a conference and can similarly improve final reporting quality by attracting widespread external review. Review comments about netprints are increasingly being posted electronically with the article. This does not replace the existing peer-review process but does provides a level of criticism that is made public. In effect, netprints have provided an opportunity for the credibility of early findings to be openly challenged prior to formal publication. It was initially hoped that electronically posted reader feedback would lead to the same kinds of benefits as the established external reviewer processes. However, in practice, the review comments are not usually as thorough as an external review and they are not confidential.

One disadvantage of netprints is that they cannot be located using standard search methods such as MEDLINE®. However, some can be found in other ways (www[7]). More importantly, studies that have a poor scientific basis and would not have been published because they did not survive the peer-review process are made public. Such studies have the potential to lead to harmful practices in patient care. It is early days for electronic publishing and many changes in the acceptability, format, and scope of e-journals and netprints can be expected in the next few years.[16]

At this time, the value of netprints to scientific advancement remains uncertain and journal editors continue to have misgivings. Although some journals will not consider accepting later versions of netprints for publication in their journal, many others will.[15-17] If your work has been posted on the web, editors will expect you to provide details of where it has been posted so that they can consider whether your paper adds new information to the medical literature. Before you consider posting your work on the web, it is prudent to investigate the copyright restrictions of the journal in which you would ultimately like to publish.

Citation index

The concept behind citation indexing is fundamentally simple. By recognising that the value of information is determined by those who use it, what better way to measure the quality of the work than by measuring the impact it makes on the community at large.

Dr Eugene Garfield (Founder and Chairman
Emeritus of ISI®)

When a journal article is cited in another journal article it earns a scientific merit point. These merit points are formally recorded in what is known as the Science Citation Index (SCI®). The Science Citation Index is a commercial database that contains information of citations from the reference lists of many published medical papers. This database is produced by the Institute for Scientific Information (ISI®) in Philadelphia (www[8]), which also produces the weekly publication *Current Contents* that lists all journal articles published in 1375 scientific journals. Records in the Science Citation Index show how many times each publication has been cited within a certain period and by whom. Thus, the citation rate of a paper can be easily calculated by counting up the number of citations it receives in the years following publication. The average citation rate per year is often regarded as a marker of the scientific merit of the article especially if the annual citation rate becomes higher than the impact factor (see p 158) of the journal.

The Science Citation Index has been printed in paper copy for many decades and citations from as early as 1945 are now available through the ISI® website. Approximately 6000 major journals are indexed in the electronic Science Citation Index and over 2100 journals are indexed in the printed copy. The electronic database is constantly updated with approximately 17 750 new records added each week. As such, it is an important log of scientific activity.

Impact factors

It is dangerous to use any kind of statistical data out of context. The use of journal impact factors as surrogates for actual citation performance is to be avoided, if at all possible.

Eugene Garfield (Founder and Chairman
Emeritus of ISI®, www.garfield.library.upenn-edu)

An impact factor is calculated as the total number of citations from a journal in one year divided by the average number of journal articles published in the previous two years and, as such, is a mean citation rate. Impact factors, which are also commercially available on the ISI® database (www[8]), have a range of 0 to 50. Examples of the impact factors of some journals are shown in Table 6.1. Whereas papers are commonly rated by their citation rates, journals are commonly rated by their impact factors. Impact factors are useful for assessing the citation rates of journals when evaluating quality or choosing a journal in which to publish.

A criticism of impact factors is that the method of calculation tends to perpetuate bias in favour of some journals.[18] In the calculation, editorials, letters, abstracts, etc. are included in the numerator but only original articles and reviews are included in the denominator. Books are not included at all but, interestingly, self-citations are. Thus, a journal that includes many editorials, letters, and reviews may have an impact factor that is inflated when compared to another journal that largely publishes original research papers. Journals that publish fewer papers have a smaller denominator and therefore tend to have a higher impact factor.

Table 6.1 Examples of the impact factors of selected journals in 2001.

Journal	Impact factor
General and multidisciplinary journals	
Nature	28·833
New England Journal of Medicine	28·660
Lancet	11·793
Annals of Internal Medicine	10·900
JAMA	9·522
BMJ	5·325
Journal of Pediatrics	3·014
Archives of Diseases in Childhood	1·712
Medical Journal of Australia	1·677
Australia and New Zealand Journal of Medicine	0·617
Clinical journals	
American Journal of Respiratory and Critical Care Medicine	5·211
Breast Cancer Research and Treatment	2·287
Obstetrics and Gynaecology	2·252
Movement Disorders	2·136
Sleep	1·880
Hormone Research	1·780
Pediatric Pulmonology	0·978
Cardiology	0·784
Medical Oncology	0·636
Specialist journals	
Advances in Cancer Research	13·250
Thorax	3·980
American Journal of Public Health	3·576
Transplantation	3·522
Journal of Nuclear Medicine	3·064
Journal of Clinical Epidemiology	1·744
Allergy	1·667
Metabolism	1·652
Journal of Inherited Metabolic Diseases	1·407
Anaesthesia and Intensive Care	0·861

The impact factor of a journal depends on the quality of the work that scientists submit to the journal and thus on the ability of a journal to attract the best papers available. Impact factors are influenced by the quality of the reviewers who help to maintain a high scientific standard. The speed of the review

Table 6.2 Grouping journals by summing five-year impact factors.[21]

Rank	Five-year impact factor index	Examples of journals
1	Below 6	*Digestion* *Gastroenterologie clinique et biologique* *Italian Journal of Gastroenterology and Hepatology* *Journal of Pediatric Gastroenterology and Nutrition*
2	From 6 to 10	*American Journal of Gastroenterology* *Clinical Science* *Journal of Hepatology* *Liver* *Scandinavian Journal of Gastroenterology*
3	From 11 to 20	*Alimentary Pharmacology & Therapeutics* *Biochemical and Biophysical Research Communications* *BMJ* *British Journal of Cancer* *Gut* *Infection and Immunity*
4	Above 20	*American Journal of Pathology* Gastroenterology *JAMA* *Lancet* *New England Journal of Medicine* *Proceedings of the National Academy of Sciences of the United States of America*

and publication processes, the content of papers and the size of the readership of the journal also have a significant influence on impact factors.[19] In many fields of research, the most cited journal articles are papers that report the development of research methods and review articles rather than papers that report original research findings. Thus, journals that favour the publication of editorials, comments, reviews, and methodological articles tend to have inherently higher impact factors.

For more than 40 years, impact factors have been used by many research institutions to rank and evaluate journals.

Many institutions also use impact factors to evaluate the merit of publications of both individual researchers and their departments. Although the quality of a paper may not necessarily agree with citation rates,[20] a better system has yet to be introduced. Table 6.2 shows an example of how journals that publish papers relevant to gastroenterology have been ranked into four categories of merit by summing the impact factors from the previous five years.[21]

The validity of an impact factor as a rating of scientific quality is often questioned. There is evidence that the journal name does not alter readers' impressions of the quality of a journal article even when they have an epidemiology or biostatistics background.[22] In addition, the mean citation rate of a journal may not be a good way to describe the average number of citations because citation rates usually have a skewed distribution with a tail towards higher rates.[18] Because this bias naturally leads to an overestimation of the average impact factor, a median would be a more appropriate statistic to use. The system has also been criticised because it heavily favours journals that are published in English and because scientists do not necessarily publish their most citable work in a journal with the highest impact factor.

It may take years for a new journal to achieve an impact factor at all. It is obviously not possible to make valid comparisons of impact factors between research fields that have different citation profiles or between journals that have different content profiles. To solve this problem, a new method of ranking journals on a percentile scale has recently been devised. The articles from over 2500 journals have now been ranked with prestige factors and, as with impact factors, the rankings are commercially available (www[9]).

In some disciplines, the quality of a journal may be determined by whether or not it is included in a subset limit of 120 "core clinical journals" within PubMed®. This listing includes journals that the National Library of Medicine in Washington, USA regards as selected biomedical journals that are of immediate interest to the practising clinician. This subset used to be known as the Abridged Index Medicus (AIM). Journals in the subset are considered to have a strict medical focus and are selected according to the quality of the journal, the usefulness of the journal content for the clinicians, and the need for providing coverage in fields of clinical medicine. Journals that are included in the subset are often ranked highly because they are considered to publish high quality papers that address important clinical issues.[23] The listing excludes "non-clinical" journals such as *Science*, *Nature*, and *Cell*.

Acknowledgements

The Bulwer-Lytton quote has been produced with permission from *Collins Concise Dictionary of Quotations, 3rd edn*. London: Harper Collins, 1998 (p 63). All other referenced quotes have been produced with permission.

Websites

1 Public Library of Science
http://www.publiclibraryofscience.org/plosjournals.htm
Publishes universally accessible and freely usable research

2 *Nature*
http://www.nature.com/nature
Publishes debate about electronic publishing

3 *Science Magazine*
http://www.sciencemag.org
Provides access to debate about electronic publishing

4 *Scientific American*
http://www.sciamcom/
Provides information about the move by scientists to publish online and the posting of published articles on the World Wide Web

5 BioMed Central
http://www.biomedcentral.com
Website at which researchers can search, read, post, or respond to non-peer-reviewed articles in the form of netprints

6 Clinical Medical and Health Research
http://clinmed.netprints.org
Website at which researchers can search, read, post, or respond to non-peer-reviewed articles in the form of netprints

7 Electronic Journal Miner
http://ejournal.coalliance.org

Website that allows you to search ejournals (both peer-reviewed and free publication)

8 Institute for Scientific Information
   http://www.isinet.com/isi
   http://wos.isiglobalnet2.com
   Information of current contents, citations and impact factors and a commercial database containing the Science Citation Index (SCI®)

9 Prestige Factor
   http://www.prestigefactor.com/biomedical.htm
   Information on percentile rankings of journal articles

References

1   Dunn I. *The writer's guide*. London: Allen and Unwin, 1999; p 9.
2   Instructions to authors. *Infection and Immunity* Jan 2000.
3   International Committee of Medical Journal Editors. Uniform requirements for manuscripts submitted to biomedical journals. *Ann Intern Med* 1997;**126**:36–47.
4   Britton J, Knox AJ. Duplicate publication, redundant publication, and disclosure of closely related articles. *Thorax* 1999;**54**:378.
5   Notice of duplicate publication. *Arch Dis Child* 2001;**85**:269.
6   Fontanarosa PB, Flanigan A. Prepublication release of medical research. *JAMA* 2000;**284**:2927–9.
7   Ellard J. How to make an editor's life easier. *Australasian Psychiatry* 2001;**9**:212–14.
8   Peat JK, Mellis CM, Williams K, Xuan W. Project management. In: *Health science research. A handbook of quantitative methods*. Melbourne: Allen and Unwin, 2001; pp 154–158.
9   Campion EW. Notification about early-release articles. *N Engl J Med* 1999;**341**:2085.
10 Voelker R. Publishers debate future of online journals. *JAMA* 2000;**284**:943–4.
11 Delamothe T, Mullner M, Smith R. Pleasing both authors and readers. *BMJ* 1999;**318**:888–9.
12 Shah S, Peat JK, Mazurski EJ, *et al*. Effect of peer led programme for asthma education in adolescents: cluster randomised controlled trial. *BMJ* 2001;**322**:583–8.
13 Delamothe T, Smith R. The joy of being electronic. *BMJ* 1999;**319**:465–6.
14 Rennie D. Freedom and responsibility in medical publication. Setting the balance right. *JAMA* 1998;**280**:300–2.
15 Delamothe T. Netprints: the next phase in the evolution of biomedical publishing. *BMJ* 1999;**319**:1515–16.
16 Smith R. Electronic publishing in science. *BMJ* 2001;**322**:627–8.
17 Smith R. Opening up *BMJ* peer review. *BMJ* 1999;**318**:4–5.
18 Seglen PO. Why the impact factors of journals should not be used for evaluating research. *BMJ* 1997;**314**:498–502.
19 Knox AJ, Britton J. Journal impact factors for 2000. *Thorax* flying yet higher. *Thorax* 2001;**56**:587.

20 Garfield E. How can impact factors be improved? *BMJ* 1996;**313**:411–13.
21 Lewison G, Grant J, Jansen P. International gastroenterology research: subject areas, impact, and funding. *Gut* 2001;**49**:295–302.
22 Christakis DA, Saint S, Saha S, *et al.* Do physicians judge a study by its cover? An investigation of journal attribution bias. *J Clin Epidemiol* 2000;**53**:773–8.
23 Greene WL, Concato J, Feinstein AR. Claims of equivalence in medical research: are they supported by the evidence? *Ann Intern Med* 2000;**132**:715–22.

7: Other types of documents

The research you have conducted is obviously of vital importance and must be read by the widest possible audience. It is probably safer to insult a colleague's spouse, family and driving than the quality of his or her research.

George Hall[1]

The objectives of this chapter are to understand how to:

- express your opinions in a letter, editorial, or narrative review
- become an author of a systematic or Cochrane review
- write a postgraduate thesis

One of the fundamental purposes of medical journals is to publish original research results in the form of journal articles. However, journals publish many other types of informative and educational items. In this chapter, we describe how to write other types of publishable documents and how to approach writing a postgraduate thesis. The writing of grant applications is also an area of scientific writing that is fundamental to research success. Many of the principles of how to write and publish journal articles described in the previous chapters apply to all of these areas of scientific writing. However, we have not included information of how to write grant applications in this book because they require a different type of attitude to scientific publications, and there are several resources that explain how to write them (www[1,2]).[2-4]

Letters

The concluding part of correspondence should not take up more than two paragraphs – one to make your point, and one to end on a pleasant note if necessary.

Elizabeth Murphy[5]

Letters, or communications as they are sometimes called, are written for many reasons. You many want to provide supporting information, clarification, criticism, correction, or an alternative explanation to the results in a previously published journal article. You may disagree with the interpretation of the results, have further information to add to a publication, or have a novel comment to make. Many journals also publish letters that convey political or psychosocial messages that are related to the practice of medicine or research.

If you decide to write a letter, it needs to carry a clear and succinct message and to have instant appeal. Only consider writing a letter if what you want to say justifies a communication. Before you begin writing, it is best to read the correspondence section of recent issues of the journal to get a feel for the type and style of letter that is published. Suggestions on how to write clear letters can be found on the web (www[3]).

Although letters are short, they often take a surprising amount of time to write, hone, and perfect. Even so, the editorial committee may edit and shorten your letter even further. However, do not rely on this. If your letter is too long, it may not be considered for publication at all and your message will not reach your audience. In most journals, letters have to conform to a word limit. For example, 500 words or two pages is usually the maximum and this may include a figure or a table. The number of authors is also usually limited to a maximum of four to six, and the number of references is usually limited to less than five including a reference to the journal article to which the letter relates.

A list of titles of letters from a single issue of *BMJ* is shown in Box 7.1. The topics are extremely varied and include comments on previous publications and news items, warnings about the safe disposal of old equipment, and the applicability of new treatment methods. The letters also include an educational note about a new website that is relevant to the health of over one billion people worldwide, and a comment on whether the term "coronary heart disease" is a tautology.

Box 7.1 Titles of letters from *BMJ* 2001; (7314) 22 Sept

Title: Duration of breastfeeding and adult arterial distensibility
Purpose: To offer criticism of the methods and interpretation of an article. Seven letters are printed under this heading plus a response from the authors. The letters editor comments that 51 responses were received of which 46 were openly critical.

Title: Debate on screening for breast cancer is not over
Purpose: To criticise the overinterpretation of a study which claimed a 63% reduction in breast cancer deaths in women screened.

Title: Mercury sphygmomanometers: disposal has far-reaching consequences
Purpose: To comment on the safe disposal of sphygmomanometers in response to an article about a trend away from their use.

Title: Risks with continuous subcutaneous insulin infusion can be serious
Purpose: To point out that although a recent editorial advocated treatment with continuous subcutaneous insulin infusion in a small proportion of diabetics, the treatment has serious risks and should not be used by physicians inexperienced in pump therapy.

Title: Islam with the internet could do much to prevent disease
Purpose: To promote an internet course of lectures on health care for Islamic people.

Title: "Coronary heart disease" is not tautologous
Purpose: To debate appropriate terms to describe disease of the heart and coronary arteries.

Most letters are written to offer criticism of a previous publication, although some offer support. If you feel the need to criticise the work of others in print, you must put forward a reasoned argument rather than make general comments. Always be polite and constructive rather than arrogant and critical. Rather than writing *Smith* et al. *were clearly wrong in their interpretation of their data*, it is better to couch this sentiment in a phrase such as *There may be another interpretation of the data presented by Smith* et al.

Remember, if your letter is published, it will remain in print a long time after your emotions have subsided. Above all else, whether you are criticising or supporting the previous work of other researchers, you must introduce a new and different perspective on the work if you want your letter to be printed.

As with other publications, letters are often treated much as original papers and sent out for external peer review. However, some journals publish non-reviewed letters that relate to matters raised in the journal in the previous six weeks. A letter in response to previously published work may be sent to the authors of the work, and your letter plus the authors' responses are then published together.

Some journals such as *BMJ* and *Archives of Diseases in Childhood* now offer a rapid response feature. This means that you can use the web to send an email response to a published paper. To send a response, log onto the paper's website, click on the journal article that you want to respond to and send an email outlining your thoughts. Provided that your response is not libellous or obscene, it will be posted on the journal website in a relatively short time, usually less than seven days. To read it, all you need to do is click on "Read rapid responses" on the homepage. As with other letters, the editors may select your letter for publication in a future paper issue.

Editorials

Writing is an exploration. You start from nothing and learn as you go.

EL Doctorow
(www.bartelby.com)

The best editorials are usually short, pithy, pertinent reviews about a topic that is selected by the editor. An editorial is often commissioned to comment on a paper that is published in the same issue of the journal. Very often, the editor asks an external reviewer who has shown insight into the paper to write this type of timely review.

Writing an editorial can be a rewarding way to disseminate your personal beliefs about a specific research area. The editorial is often more far reaching than a journal article because researchers are more likely to read it and because you have the opportunity to extend thinking beyond simply interpreting the study results. It is always exciting to be asked to write an editorial but if you accept the challenge, be sure that you have some new insights into the subject matter and that you can complete the task before the set deadline. Journals will not want to delay the publication of a paper because the editorial is not ready and for this reason usually ask authors to sign a binding contract.

If you are asked to write an editorial but do not have broad expertise in the research area, it is usually acceptable to enrol coauthors. Writers often enrol coauthors with specific expert experience. If as an epidemiologist you are asked to write an editorial about the effects of breastfeeding, you will probably want to enrol an expert in early infant feeding. If as an expert in early infant feeding, you are asked to write an editorial about a population study of breastfeeding, you will probably want to enrol an epidemiologist. As a result, the article will be more grounded and fully informed than if you had written it by yourself.

Writing an editorial does not require you to provide any original study results but it does require you to make judgements on the basis of a selective review of the literature. Because medical research has been heavily supported by the pharmaceutical industry, it is important that the opinions expressed in editorials are independent of any types of financial influence. Thus, it is important that editorial authors do not have any financial ties to companies that manufacture any products that are discussed[6] and, to circumvent this, editorial writers are often asked to make strict declarations of any conflicts of interest.

Narrative reviews

In the writing process, the more a story cooks, the better.

Doris Lessing
(www.bartelby.com)

Review articles are very popular with readers and editors. Very short reviews are often called annotations. Editors like reviews because they know that, along with the editorials and the correspondence columns, they are the most widely read part of a scientific journal.[7] To maintain reader interest, review articles must be topical, up to date, accurate and authoritative, and, if possible, provocative and a good read.

Narrative reviews are usually written to address new developments or to summarise recent literature on a topic of wide interest to clinicians or researchers. Editors usually commission authors who are considered to be experts in their fields of research. Although many reviews are written at the invitation of editorial committees and may bring an honorarium payment, unsolicited reviews may also be accepted. Journals such as the *BMJ* forward-plan forthcoming theme issues that are selected by both a readers' poll and the editorial committee.[8] For such issues, the editorials and other educational articles are commissioned by the editors. However, if you have an issue that you would like to write about, you can approach the editors and put your suggestions to them.

Some examples of titles of annotations and reviews are shown in Box 7.2. As discussed in Chapter 4, titles for reviews benefit from being short, catchy, and humorous if possible.

Box 7.2 Titles of annotations and reviews

Bugs and the gut: breaking barriers[9]
Perinatal pathology in 2001[10]
The diagnosis of Prader–Willi syndrome[11]
Suffocation, shaking, or sudden infant death: can we tell the difference?[12]
Folate before pregnancy: are we doing enough?[13]
Prion proteins and the gut: une liaison dangereuse?[14]
Rett syndrome: clinical update and review of recent genetics advances[15]
Beds, bedroom, bedding, and bugs: anything new between the sheets?[16]
Similar, the same, or just not different: a guide for deciding whether treatments are clinically equivalent[17]
Of mice, men, and microbes: hantavirus[18]

When you are reading the literature, remember that reviews published in journal supplements may be of inferior quality to reviews published in the parent journal. Most journal supplements are commercially sponsored and the articles may not undergo external peer review.[19]

If you are contracted to write a review, consider the length of the final document and the time you will need to research the content. Do not underestimate the time it will take to access and digest the relevant information. Also consider whether the topic is something that you find important and exciting, and whether you have new insights that readers will find novel or inspiring. If you are not certain that you have anything new to say or that you can deliver the review on time, do not be tempted to accept the contract. It will not improve your reputation if you sign the contract and then either fail to meet the deadline or produce an inferior product.

Writing a narrative review does not constrain you to sections of the literature as would writing a systematic review. It is generally accepted that narrative reviews are an expert opinion that is an extension of current thinking and not a definitive evaluation of the literature. However, narrative reviews should always be based on the most recent knowledge and the most rigorous evidence. If you want to extend thinking and influence future research directions, you must base your opinions on the best evidence available.

Narrative reviews have sometimes been criticised as "old fashioned" because they do not need to specify a search strategy, the criteria for inclusion and exclusion of studies, or the way in which the quality of citations was assessed. Bias can be introduced if all relevant studies including those that are unpublished or in a foreign language are not identified. Bias can also be introduced by the overuse of the authors' own studies or studies that support their viewpoints, the exclusion of studies with negative results, and the preferential selection of studies with which the authors are familiar. For this reason, some journals now require that the search strategy and inclusion criteria for publications are stated clearly in narrative reviews.

Writing a narrative review can sometimes seem a daunting process but, as shown in Box 7.3, there are some ways to ease the process. A divide and conquer approach is best. Once you have divided up the tasks involved into smaller, manageable pieces, and approached them in a sequential order, writing the review becomes simpler, more purposeful, and more organised. You should outline your topic at the beginning of the review and come to some clear conclusions or recommendations at the end. Reviews take less time to write and are more rewarding to write if you begin with an organised plan.

Box 7.3 Sequential steps for writing a narrative review

Make decisions about novel ideas or new opinions around which the review will be centred
Decide on a literature search strategy
Collect all relevant literature
Enrol coauthors if necessary
Enter citations into an electronic database
Organise journal articles into groups that will form subheadings
Within subheadings, organise literature into subgroups that form topic sentences
Fill in the content
Ask for peer review from a variety of people
Update with any newly published literature or new ideas as you progress

---

If you have in mind a review that you would like to write and think a journal may be interested, it is a good idea to approach the editor before you begin writing. You should explain how long you expect the review and the citation list to be and when you expect the review to be ready for submission. In general, brief reviews take priority for publication over lengthy reviews. It is not a good idea to begin writing a review if you are not sure where it will be published. If the journal is not interested in the topic you have chosen, you will be disappointed, but at least you won't have wasted time writing something that is unlikely to be published.

Systematic reviews and Cochrane reviews

It is surely a great criticism of our profession that we have not organised a critical summary, by specialty or sub-specialty adapted periodically, of all relevant randomised controlled trials.

Archie Cochrane[20]

Systematic reviews are a more rigorous compilation of evidence from the literature than narrative reviews simply because the search strategy for finding and summarising studies is clearly defined. In a systematic review of the literature, all of the primary studies on a topic are systematically identified, critically appraised, and summarised, with explicit and reproducible methods. The rationale behind this approach is that the standardisation and the transparency of the methods used by authors and the acquisition of all available primary studies on the review topic minimise the potential for bias.

A systematic review conducted under the guidance of the Cochrane Collaboration is naturally known as a Cochrane review. These reviews, which are named after Archie Cochrane who was an epidemiologist in the late 1970s, are high quality systematic reviews that provide substantial evidence that is relevant to health care. To date over 1000 reviews and 800 protocols for reviews are collated in the Cochrane Library.[21] The library, which is available on CD or through the web (www[4]), contains the Cochrane Database of Systematic Reviews (CDSR). The library also contains the Database of Abstracts of Reviews of Effectiveness (DARE) that includes abstracts of systematic reviews conducted outside the Cochrane Collaboration but deemed to be of high quality.

Authors who would like to conduct a systematic review for publication in the CDSR must first register their title with a Cochrane Collaborative review group and then submit a protocol to them. Protocols must include the review objectives, search strategy, criteria for inclusion and exclusion of studies, and information of the types of outcome measures to be obtained. Submitted protocols are reviewed by the Cochrane Collaboration to eliminate any methodological flaws before the protocol is accepted and included in the CDSR. Once the protocol is accepted, the extraction and summary of data can be undertaken.

Guidelines for writing and formatting Cochrane reviews are available at the Cochrane website (www[5]). Data extraction from primary studies must be conducted independently by at least two reviewers with contentious issues being resolved by a third party. Software called Review Manager® (RevMan) has been developed to help authors prepare reviews in a standardised format and can also be obtained from the Cochrane website (www[6]).

The components of a Cochrane review are shown in Box 7.4. When the review is published on the CDSR, comments and criticisms in the form of electronic letters are linked to it and any ensuing changes are also published.[22] This process leads to a continual updating and correction of any errors or potential biases.

Box 7.4 Format of a Cochrane review

Cover sheet

Title, citation, contact reviewer, other authors, and contact addresses, date of latest substantive update, details of contributions made by all individuals who contributed to the review, sources of support

Synopsis

Abstract

Structured format

Text of review

Introduction including background, objectives
Materials and methods including study selection criteria, study types, participants or population, interventions, outcome measures, and search strategy
Results including study description, methodological quality, and individual results
Discussion
Conclusions

Tables and figures

Characteristics of studies included/excluded/ongoing
Details of interventions that were compared
Results of studies included/excluded/ongoing
Meta-analysis graphs

References

Details of the included, excluded, and ongoing studies

Comments and criticisms

Cochrane reviews have a structured abstract of up to 400 words. This is a stand-alone document that gives details of the background, objectives, search strategy, selection criteria, data collection and analysis, main results, and reviewers' conclusions. Most Cochrane reviews address a question of

General elderly people

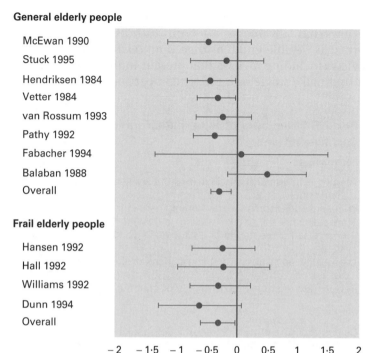

Figure 7.1 Effectiveness of home based support for older people: systematic review and meta-analysis. Produced with permission from R Elkan *et al. BMJ* 2001;**323**:719.[23]

therapy and thus are reviews of randomised or quasi-randomised controlled trials. In some reviews, results are summarised using a meta-analysis that is a statistical method for combining the results from several studies. The software Review Manager® (RevMan) is used to undertake the meta-analyses and present the results in a standard graphical format. An example of summarising results in a single figure is shown in Figure 7.1.

The publication of a Cochrane review in the Cochrane Library does not prevent you from also publishing the review in an abbreviated form in a peer-reviewed journal. However, writing a Cochrane review is an ongoing responsibility because authors are expected to update their review on an annual basis.

As shown in Box 7.5, the standard format of Cochrane reviews has advantages to both authors and readers. The format is flexible enough to accommodate different types of reviews including reviews that present individual patient data or that make single or multiple comparisons.

Box 7.5 Advantages of using a standard format for Cochrane reviews

For readers

The title is informative and identifies the problem addressed and the intervention

Summarised research results from primary studies are easy to find

Standardised headings allow readers to find the information of interest

Standardised presentation of results ensures comparability between studies

The validity, applicability, and implications of the results are easy to assess

Reviews are easy to read on screen or print out

For authors

Guides explicit and concise reporting of results

Minimises effort of reporting

Suitable for electronic submission for review and publishing

Allows for updating

Role of authors and contributors is clearly identified

Despite the rigorous methods and peer-review processes, a recent audit of Cochrane reviews published in 1998 found some limitations. In some reviews, the reporting was unsatisfactory or the conclusion was not supported by the evidence.[22] Since 1998, the Cochrane Collaboration has undertaken additional steps to avoid problems such as these and thus to improve review quality. With continual updates to the review handbook, errors in reviews will continue to be reduced and Cochrane reviews will maintain their place as the least biased of all types of reviews.

Case reports

Case reporting is arguably the oldest and most basic form of communication in medicine.

JAW Wildsmith[24]

Most clinical journals publish case reports that explain how patients presented for medical care, how the course of the illness progressed, and what treatment was given. Case reports that publish this information for a number of patients are called case series. The main purpose of a case report is to educate clinicians about the clinical features, investigation, and/or the treatment of patients with unusual problems. A case report often acts as refresher training for clinicians so that a diagnosis is made more readily and the condition treated more effectively. In reporting observations by clinicians, case reports may also generate hypotheses that lead to new research studies. The topics that are often the subject of case reports are shown in Box 7.6.

Box 7.6 Topics that may be reported in case reports

Clinical conditions that have not been described before
Unusual and unreported presentations of known clinical conditions
Unexpected beneficial responses to a treatment
Previously unreported adverse reactions to a treatment
Errors in diagnosis as a result of use of incorrect tests or presentation with unusual symptoms
New uses of a diagnostic tool or use of novel diagnostic tools
Phenotypes associated with a newly found gene

Whatever the topic, case reports need to provide new information. For example, the journal *Gut* welcomes "case reports of outstanding interest or clinical relevance" but specifies that such reports "should include a significant scientific advance in our understanding of disease aetiology or pathogenetic mechanisms." Because styles of case reports vary widely it is prudent to check the instructions to authors (www[7]) before beginning to write a report.

Most journals restrict the size of case reports. For example, *Gut* restricts reports to 1500 words, 15 references, one table and two figures; the *Journal of Pediatric Gastroenterology and Nutrition* restricts reports to eight manuscript pages including any figures, tables, and references. Sometimes an illustrative case report may be reported in the context of a literature review. However, because the main purpose of most case reports is simply to describe the patient and any relevant features, there is usually no need for a literature review in either the introduction or discussion sections.

The *New England Journal of Medicine* publishes different types of case reports. One to three cases of a condition can be described in a brief report with a maximum of 2000 words, but clinical problem-solving reports are larger with a maximum of 2500 words and 20 references. These reports may include imaging and pathology results, presented in stages in order to replicate the way in which information was obtained in clinical practice. Reports that discuss different diagnoses in the context of the pathophysiology of the patient often provide useful teaching material. Selected case reports together with medical images and a medical quiz are available at the web site (www[8]).

Whatever the format of a case report it is important to ensure that the patient is described as a person and not as a case. Patient anonymity must be maintained at all times and any names on test results or images must be blacked out. Consent for the use of clinical photographs should always be obtained from the patient themselves or from the parents or guardians of children.

Postgraduate theses

Planning to write is about writing. Outlining ... researching ... talking to people about what you're doing, none of that is writing. Writing is writing.

EL Doctorow
(www.bartelby.com)

Postgraduate theses, whether they are for a doctorate or masters degree, command a huge time and emotional commitment. The required length of a postgraduate thesis may vary widely but, for a doctorate, the range is generally 35 000–50 000 words with an upper limit often set at 80 000 words. If you are unsure how long your thesis should be, check with your institutional guidelines. Whether 40 000 or 80 000 words are used, writing a thesis is a long and daunting task and it may not become satisfying until the end is in sight. However, if you write with a plan in mind, the process will be more rewarding.

When you begin a postgraduate degree, it is important to have a clear idea of your own responsibilities in addition to those of your supervisors and your institution. Most institutions publish a code of practice for the supervision of postgraduate research students that outlines the responsibilities of the institution, the department, the supervisor, and the candidate. The codes are quite detailed and are designed to ensure that candidates receive the support and educational facilities that they need. In return, candidates should be prepared to establish working guidelines with their supervisor and to execute their project within the time-lines defined. Before you begin your degree, it is a good idea to familiarise yourself with the codes of practice at your institution.

As a research student, it will be your responsibility to negotiate what your thesis will contain, to write the thesis, and to submit it for examination. In many institutions, the award of your degree will depend entirely on your thesis, and therefore it is important that it is self-contained, conveys your competency and demonstrates an original contribution to knowledge. If you are having problems writing your thesis, you may benefit from accessing online information (www[9-11]) or from joining or forming a writers group as discussed in Chapter 12. Attending and presenting your results at scientific meetings often provides inspiration and a valuable peer-review process. Also, regular attendance at journal clubs will help you to keep up to date with the literature and appraise new journal articles correctly.

The steps to writing a literature review for a postgraduate thesis are shown in Box 7.7. Often, the literature review is one of the most burdensome parts to write. An effective way to summarise the literature is often to log the results from all relevant studies into a table/tables that you update regularly.

Box 7.7 Writing a literature review for a postgraduate thesis

Organise your thoughts in a logical order
Use headings to create major sections that deal with different topics
Use subheadings to guide your readers and examiners
Use graphs, tables, and diagrams to summarise or highlight information
Finish with a summary of the major points
Identify the limitations of published studies
Raise questions that you will answer in your thesis
Leave the reader wanting to know what the answer will be

Your literature review is in effect a narrative review and can be constructed using the guidelines for a narrative review that were shown in Box 7.3. Because the literature reviews from postgraduate theses are often published as narrative reviews, it may help to write it with this idea in mind.

Remember that you can often be more expansive in your thesis than you would be if writing for a journal. The main purpose of your literature review is to provide a background for your work. You may like to put your research in a historical context, summarise all of the relevant work to date, including a critique of the strengths and weaknesses of previous studies, and raise any questions that you plan to address in your thesis. You must also be prepared to continue to update and rewrite your review as your study and candidature evolve. Although you can start on your literature review at the beginning of your candidature and develop it as you progress, you can only finalise this section once you are certain of the outcome of your research work.

The typical contents of a postgraduate thesis are shown in Box 7.8. When you begin to write your thesis, you need to create a document with these titles as chapter headings with each on a new page. Under each heading or subheading, you can make notes or add text, results, and references. If you can just write a paragraph or two at a time, your aim is no longer a thesis, which is a daunting goal, but is something much simpler and achievable. By using this divide and conquer approach, you will avoid some of the issues of writer's block. Completing a few sections will give you the confidence to fill in all of the remaining sections.

Box 7.8 Typical contents of a postgraduate thesis

Title page
Declaration
Ethics clearances
Acknowledgements
Abstract
Table of contents
Lists of figures and tables
Publications arising (papers and abstracts)

List of abbreviations
Introduction
Aims and/or hypotheses
Literature review
Methods
Results chapters
Discussion
Conclusions and future directions
References
Appendices

Much of the body of the thesis can be put together using the guidelines for writing a journal article that are discussed in previous chapters and the writing style that is described in later chapters. If your thesis is written to the high standard that is acceptable for publishing a paper in a well-respected journal, then it will also be written to appeal to your supervisors and markers. However, in a thesis you can provide a little more detail than you would for a journal article. Also, you need to follow through so that each chapter leads into the next. Keep reminding yourself that it doesn't matter if it doesn't hang together perfectly at the beginning. You will be able to shape your thesis into a coherent story at the end, especially if you have been conducting your research using a well-organised plan.

Format of a postgraduate thesis

I just sit at the typewriter and curse a bit.

PG Wodehouse
(www.bartelby.com)

You will have started your research with aims and/or hypotheses that may have been modified during the course of your candidature. A useful way of presenting your thesis is to have a small introductory chapter that outlines the main aims and hypotheses of the research work that you are presenting. This section may be no more than two pages in length, but it will set the scene for the remainder of the thesis and will orientate your examiners to what your work is all about.

The format and structure in which you write your literature review can vary widely. Some postgraduate theses have a major literature review at the beginning and then smaller reviews at the start of each results chapter. Other postgraduate students choose to have a single major literature review with a very brief introduction at the start of each results chapter. It is up to you and your supervisor to decide which approach is most appropriate for the work that you are undertaking.

Your methods and results sections should be the "meat" of your thesis. Some researchers present a large methods chapter with clear information about each technique used followed by several results chapters. In this case, each results chapter answers a separate research question but refers back, as needed, to the methods section. An alternative approach is to write a methods section that is relevant to all chapters and then include methods that are unique to each research question within each chapter. At the extreme, a main methods section may be absent and each results chapter will contain its own methods. It is essential to choose a style that best fits the studies that you will conduct and try not to alter the style too many times as you progress.

In writing your discussion and conclusions sections, there are two approaches that can be used. Each results chapter can have a very detailed discussion and you can include a relatively brief conclusions chapter to highlight the main points. Alternatively, each results chapter can include some discussion and then you need to provide a more detailed and reasonably lengthy discussion in the formal discussion and conclusions chapters. The approach that you take will, again, depend on the types of studies that you have conducted but, whatever approach you adopt, you must ensure that your conclusions match up with the initial aims and/or hypotheses that you outlined in the introduction. Ensure that you bring all of your findings together in a final section that leaves the examiners in no doubt about the importance and applicability of your work.

Most postgraduate theses have appendices that list information that is not germane to the main flow of the research work but helps readers and examiners to understand the methods and results more fully. The type of information that is included in the appendices may be questionnaires that were used, consent forms, mathematical derivations of equations used, raw data, etc. This information is included for completeness and for other researchers who may want to refer to the details at a later date. It is unlikely that examiners will read this section, so do not file any information in the appendices that is essential to the interpretation of your results.

Tips for completing a postgraduate thesis

Writing is like carrying a fetus.

Edna O'Brien
(www.bartelby.com)

Box 7.9 Tips for writing a postgraduate thesis

Start with a firm plan in mind and have clear aims that you will address

Keep your literature review up to date

Set a time-line for completion and ensure that it is appropriate for the aims

Review the broad outline of your thesis regularly

Identify the people who are responsible for different aspects of your postgraduate experience

Make a timetable that defines how much regular contact you will have with your supervisor/s

Forward plan appointments with supervisors and stick to them

Write up your methods section as you go

Complete the process sections of your thesis as early as possible including the ethics declarations, list of abbreviations, appendices, and acknowledgements

Write the first draft of each section as soon as you can

Refine draft chapters and pass each one to your supervisor/s as you progress

Elicit peer review from many different sources including friendly "experts", fellow students, postdoctoral fellows, friends, and family

Be specific and ask for macro-feedback on content or micro-feedback on the presentation, writing style, and grammar

Give your reviewers plenty of time to read drafts and provide comments

Attend all educational seminars and training sessions that you can

Present your results at local, national, and international scientific meetings

Set a time-line for submission

Publish results chapters as journal articles as you proceed

Some tips for writing a thesis are shown in Box 7.9. As a postgraduate student, you should have the benefit of being able to obtain peer review and expertise easily from your supervisors and collaborators, and this should provide a substantial foundation for your work. Ideally, you will have one or more mentors as discussed in Chapter 12. However, you are responsible for writing your thesis and for ensuring that it receives adequate peer review as you progress. Thus, it is important to complete your thesis in small sections to avoid passing large sections or even the entire thesis to your supervisors for comment. You must also give your reviewers ample time to read and digest what you have written – one to two weeks for each chapter is a minimum and many reviewers may take longer. By planning an adequate review process, you will ensure that you treat your reviewers with respect and that you receive the highest quality feedback that is possible.

It is important that you have a broad educational focus as a postgraduate student. To facilitate learning, you must attend any courses that are relevant to you and present your work widely. Presenting your data at a scientific meeting often helps to clarify thinking and may result in helpful feedback from experts in your field. If you can publish some of your chapters as journal articles as you go, this will send a message to your examiners that you have survived an external peer-review process and that your work has been considered worthy of publication. In this situation, examiners will be more likely to regard your work favourably and will be unable to reject your thesis easily.

Your institution, postgraduate office, or supervisor will have specific guidelines to help you write your postgraduate thesis to the standard required and to deal with the submission and marking processes. You will need to be aware of the maximum thesis length and the necessary margin sizes, spacing, font size, etc. It is a good idea to look at previous theses that are held in university libraries or archives and to talk with other postgraduate students. You will also need to familiarise yourself with the submission and marking system so that you do not unnecessarily delay submission, and so that you have a realistic expectation of the time that it may take before you receive a decision from the markers and your postgraduate committee.

Once your thesis is marked, you may be asked to make some amendments and these may be assessed by the postgraduate committee or sent back to the examiners for consideration. For some postgraduate degrees, there is no scope for modification and resubmission, so that your thesis has to be "perfect" the first time around. The marking system can be quite complex before the exam process is finalised. To avoid disappointment or unexpected delays, it is a good idea to ask your supervisor to explain the system that is used at your institution.

Acknowledgements

All referenced quotes have been produced with permission.

Websites

1 Learner Associates
   http://www.learnerassociates.net/proposal/
   Access to the documents "Guide for writing a funding proposal" by Dr J Levine, Michigan State University

2 Faculty of Education, University of Sydney
   http://www.edfac.usyd.edu.au/research/resource.html
   Links to various websites around the world that give tips for writing grant proposals

3 Plain English Campaign
   http://www.plainenglish.co.uk
   Guides to writing medical information including letters and reports

4 Cochrane Collaboration
   http://www.cochrane.org
   Access to Cochrane reviews

5 Cochrane Collaboration
   http://www.update-software.com/ccweb/cochrane/hbook.html
   Guidelines for authors and contributors for preparing systematic reviews of the effects of health care interventions

6 Cochrane Collaboration
   http://www.cochrane.org/cochrane/revman.html
   Access to the Cochrane Collaboration's program RevMan for preparing and maintaining Cochrane reviews

7 Medical College of Ohio, Raymon H. Mulford Library
   http://www.mco.edu/lib/instr/libinsta.html
   Links to websites that provide instructions to authors for over 2000 journals in the health sciences

8 *New England Journal of Medicine*
   http://ww.nejm.org/wtd/
   http://www.nejm.org/icm/

Access to case reports and educational "What's the diagnosis" and "Clinical Medicine Quiz" sites

9   Australasian Society for Medical Research
    http://www.asmr.org.au/conferences/thesis.html
    Guide to how to prepare a postgraduate thesis

10 Learner Associates
    http://www.learnerassociates.net/dissthes/
    Access to the document "Writing and presenting your thesis or dissertation" by Dr J Levine, Michigan State University

11 University of New South Wales, School of Physics
    http://www.phys.unsw.edu.au/~jw/thesis.html
    Access to "How to write a PhD thesis" by Joe Wolfe

References

1   Hall GM. Structure of a scientific paper. In: *How to write a paper*. London: BMJ Books, 1994; pp 1–5.
2   Crombie IK, du Florey CV. *The pocket guide to grant applications*. London: BMJ Books, 1998.
3   Goldblatt D. How to get a grant funded. *BMJ* 1998;**317**:1647–8.
4   Peat JK, Mellis CM, Williams K, Xuan W. Grantsmanship. In: *Health science research. A handbook of quantitative methods*. London: Allen and Unwin, 2001; pp 278–82.
5   Murphy E. *Effective writing: plain English at work*. Melbourne: Pitman, 1989; p 131.
6   Angell M, Kassirer JP. Editorials and conflicts of interest. *N Engl J Med* 1996;**335**:1055–6.
7   Strunin L. How to write a review. In: *How to write a paper*. Hall GM, ed. London: BMJ Books, 1994; pp 71–7.
8   Delamothe T. Forthcoming issues and how we chose them. *BMJ* 2001;**323**:766.
9   Borriello P. Bugs and the gut: breaking barriers to understanding. *Gut* 2001;**48**:443–7.
10 Cox P, Scott R. Perinatal pathology in 2001. *Arch Dis Child* 2001;**84**:457–8.
11 Smith A. The diagnosis of Prader–Willi Syndrome. *J Pediatr Child Health* 1999;**35**:335–7.
12 Byard RW, Krons HF. Suffocation, shaking or sudden infant death: can we tell the difference? *J Pediatr Child Health* 1999;**35**:432–3.
13 Bower C, Werler MM. Folate before pregnancy: are we doing enough? *Med J Aust* 2001;**174**:619–20.
14 Shmakov AN, Ghosh S. Prion proteins and the gut: une liaison dangereuse? *Gut* 2001;**35**:419–26.
15 Ellaway C, Christodoulou J. Rett syndrome: cinical update and review of recent genetics advances. *J Pediatr Child Health* 1999;**35**:419–26.
16 Siebers RW, Fitzharris P, Crane J. Beds, bedroom, bedding and bugs: anything new between the sheets? *Clin Exp Allergy* 1996;**26**:1225–7.
17 Massel D. Similar, the same or just not different: a guide for deciding whether treatments are clinically equivalent. *Can J Cardiol* 1999;**15**:556–62.

18 Book review. Of mice, men and microbes: hantavirus (letter). *N Engl J Med* 2000;**342**:666.
19 Ellard J. How to make an editor's life easier. *Australasian Psychiatry* 2001;**9**:212–14.
20 Cochrane AL. *Effectiveness and efficiency. Random reflections on health services.* London: Nuffield Provincial Hospitals Trust, 1972.
21 Clarke M, Langhorne P. Revisiting the Cochrane Collaboration. *BMJ* 2001;**323**:821.
22 Olsen O, Middleton P, Ezzo J, *et al.* Quality of Cochrane reviews: assessment of sample from 1998. *BMJ* 2001;**323**:829–32.
23 Elkan R, Kendrick D, Dewey M, *et al.* Effectiveness of home based support for older people: systematic review and meta-analysis. *BMJ* 2001;**323**:719.
24 Goldsmith JAW. How to write a case report. In: *How to write a paper.* London: BMJ Books, 1997; pp 64–70.

8: Writing style

There are two good reasons why it is desirable to write clearly: first, to be sure that you yourself know what you mean and second, to be sure that you get your message across to your readers.

Mimi Zeiger[1]

The objectives of this chapter are to understand how to:

- begin each paragraph with a purpose
- understand the basic format of sentences
- achieve clarity, brevity, and precision in your writing
- create an easily readable paper
- avoid common problems in sentence construction

The style in which you write and present your paper is of fundamental importance for achieving brevity and clarity. To convey messages effectively in written form, it is essential to have organisation both between and within your paragraphs. In this chapter, we outline some tips of how to achieve this. Further resources on how to write clearly and effectively and educational material additional to the information presented in the following chapters can be found on the web (www[1-5]).

Plain English

Prose – like food – is more easily taken in small bits.

Australian Government Publishing Service[2]

Plain English is "the art of using language that the intended audience can understand and act upon from a single reading" (www[3]). This concept has been widely adopted by many government and legal organisations, and, in some countries, new laws must now be drafted in plain English. At Cambridge University, there is even a Professor of Plain English. The Plain English Campaign that began in 1979 has promoted the use of crystal clear language and campaigned against jargon, gobbledygook, and other confusing language. The campaign also recognises that appearance matters and that the design, typeface, and layout of a paper can be as important as the language for conveying meaning. The campaign website provides free guides to plain English, details of training courses and a range of example material including a collection of gobbledygook entitled "Utter drivel". The website also includes advice about scientific writing. In the following sections, we outline our own tips and examples of how to write in plain English.

Topic sentences

> *Effective writing is writing that works. It does the job without anyone having to ask for further explanation. If it informs, it does so clearly – the reader does not have to ask for more information.*

Elizabeth Murphy[3]

Before you begin writing a paragraph, you must have a clear concept of what it is going to be about. A paragraph can be beautifully constructed but can be difficult to understand if it is not organised around a defined topic. Organising your thoughts in each paragraph can be easily achieved by using a topic sentence. Topic sentences begin a paragraph and explain what it will be about. The topic sentence creates the expectation of what the paragraph will be about and the supporting sentences fulfil that expectation.[4] For this reason, topic sentences are an essential tool for organising paragraphs and for improving the readability of your paper. Once the topic sentence has been correctly framed, the paragraph is completed with supporting sentences that give all the remaining information that the reader needs to know. Topic sentences are especially useful for writing the introduction and discussion and, to an extent, the results section. In the methods and abstract, the standard subheadings tend to replace the need for topic sentences.

If a paragraph begins with a clear topic sentence, you immediately get a good idea of what information will follow. For example, a sentence such as *Enterovirus infections in the neonatal period are common and are associated with significant morbidity and mortality* makes the paragraph content clear.[5] If you cannot write in one clear sentence what your paragraph is going to be about, then perhaps you do not need to include the paragraph at all. If you have multiple messages in your paragraph, you will need to deconstruct it into multiple paragraphs or tie the messages together in a single theme. Box 8.1 shows how the topic sentence, which is underlined, summarises the context of the paragraph and is followed by a number of sentences that support it.

Box 8.1 Example of writing a paragraph by using topic sentence followed by supporting sentences

It is unlikely that bias or confounding would account for a large proportion of the clinically important differences that we found between our study groups. The participants were selected randomly from the electoral role, we achieved a high response rate, and we used objective measurements to collect our main outcome data. Although, for safety reasons, our observers could not be blinded to the health status of the participants, objective measurements are more reliable than self-reported symptom history that is subject to recall bias. Moreover, by using multivariate analyses, we were able to adjust for any effects of major confounders. In these ways, we were able to minimise selection bias and measurement error, and we were able to control for confounding.

Topic sentences not only let the reader know what a paragraph is about but also force you, as a writer, to organise your material logically. In organising your ideas into separate thoughts and in writing topic sentences to describe the content of your paragraphs, you instil a clear and purposeful structure to your writing. Topic sentences are like mini-subheadings that act as signposts to direct readers to the part of the journal article that they are trying to find. Simply by scanning down the topic sentences, you should be able to see what information is contained in the section. Organising a paper in this standard pattern is akin to taking your reader by the hand and leading them through your thoughts. Box 8.2 shows the topic sentences in the order presented from the paragraphs of a discussion section. By scanning down the topic sentences you get a clear idea of the main issues that are discussed.

Box 8.2 Example of topic sentences adapted from a discussion section[6]

This study has important implications for both the prevention and treatment of asthma.

To estimate allergen exposures, we analysed dust from homes using an immunoassay that is sensitive and specific for measuring housedust mite allergens.

The data from the current studies add strength to the evidence that there is a causal relation between housedust mites and asthma.

We have been able to evaluate the independent effects of exposure to housedust mites by presenting the data as adjusted odds ratios that take account of sensitisation to other common allergens.

The evidence that housedust mite allergens have an important association with asthma morbidity continues to accumulate.

There is encouraging evidence that reduction of housedust mite allergen exposure can reduce asthma morbidity.

Because the prevalence of asthma has increased substantially in recent years, it is important that all avenues of preventing asthma are explored.

Subjects, verbs, and objects

Drama is life with the dull bits cut out.

Alfred Hitchcock (1899–1980)

The simplest and most easily understood sentences are constructed in a subject–verb–object format. The subject is a noun or noun cluster that begins the sentence and the object is the noun or noun cluster that ends the sentence. The two parts are then joined by a verb or verb cluster in the centre. If we take the sentence *However, cases are difficult to ascertain through retrospective population studies*, you will see that this is made up of a conjunction (*However*), a subject (*cases*), a verb cluster (*are difficult to ascertain*) and an object (*through retrospective population studies*) that is a noun cluster. Similarly, the sentence *Hospital statistics show that respiratory infections occur mostly in winter*, has a subject (*hospital statistics*), a verb (*show*) and an object (*that respiratory infections occur mostly in winter*). Both the subject and object are noun clusters.

It is important to understand this construction for analysing sentences to make them work better and flow together nicely. Of course adjectives, adjectival phrases, and clauses can be thrown in, but, if you deviate too far from the *subject–verb–object* format, your sentence will be weighed down by too many messages. Sentences become more complicated when they are made up of two simple sentences strung together or when additional phrases and clauses are added to make a compound sentence. The construction of these types of sentences is discussed in more detail in the following chapters.

Eliminating fog

> *One of the really bad things you can do to your writing is to dress up the vocabulary, looking for long words because you're maybe a little bit ashamed of the short ones. This is like dressing up a pet in evening clothes.*
>
> Stephen King[7]

It is essential to eliminate any fog, which is the dubious art of using vague thoughts and woolly words rather than short, direct ones. You can minimise fog by keeping every sentence simple and by saying exactly what you mean. To do this, you need to analyse each sentence, eliminate the unnecessary phrases and inspect the words that you have chosen.

Non-foggy writing means using simple sentences without jargon and with as few words, phrases, and clauses as possible. Readers do not want to read sentences over and over again or go in search of further information before they understand what you were trying to tell them. Few readers enjoy sifting through poor writing, pondering over ambiguities, and vainly trying to work out what they think you thought when you committed your words to paper.

Eliminating foggy writing has many benefits. The most fundamental benefit will be that you clarify your own thinking. At the beginning, you may think that you know what you want to say, but writing it down clearly can be hard. However, by working through your thoughts and by putting them in writing, you should quickly discover what you want to say and why. You may also discover that you have some inconsistencies in thinking and some incoherent ideas. In trying to write without fog, you will clarify your own ideas and be able to express what you mean more clearly to others.

You need to ensure that you do not confuse your reader by writing ambiguous sentences or by writing sentences that do not reach a proper conclusion. These types of sentences leave the reader's thoughts in mid-air.

To eliminate fog, you need to remove any fuzzy writing and unnecessary jargon. Box 8.3 shows some examples of taking the "fog" out of a sentence. In the first example, the word count is reduced from 39 to 28 words, a 28% reduction, and in the second example from 40 to 35 words. By eliminating the fog, the meaning of the sentence becomes much clearer. In the third example, the two long word clusters can be written more directly. In the fourth example, 15 words (43% of the original sentence) are removed to achieve a short, clear sentence. In examples five and six, 57% and 31% of words are removed respectively. In all examples, the corrected sentence is shorter and more direct.

Most of us can think more clearly if we have to explain a concept to another person in verbal rather than in written form. If you are unsure of what you are trying to write, it is best to leave the keyboard and find someone with whom you can discuss your thoughts. Alternatively, try closing your eyes

Box 8.3 Eliminating fog (shown underlined)

1 ✖ Bias <u>is likely to occur</u> if <u>the only</u> subjects <u>who are enrolled are those</u> who are chosen <u>specifically on</u> the basis of the presence or absence of disease so that potentially "false positive" or "false negative" cases are excluded.

   ✓ Bias can occur if participants are chosen on the basis of the presence or absence of disease so that potential "false positive" or "false negative" cases are excluded.

2 ✖ Although adults with severe obesity reported more <u>symptoms of</u> wheeze and shortness of breath, this was not associated with <u>an increase in</u> the prevalence of atopy or AHR suggesting that <u>the prevalence of asthma is not increased in this group</u>.

   ✓ Although severely obese adults experienced more wheeze and shortness of breath, this was not associated with a higher prevalence of atopy or AHR, suggesting that this group does not have a higher prevalence of asthma.

3 ✖ Observer variation <u>is due to the inability</u> of researchers to <u>administer tests in a standardised way</u>.

   ✓ Observer variation is caused by differences in the ways in which researchers collect data.

4 ✖ <u>In considering diseases that might be ameliorated by gene therapy, a setting in which</u> a selective advantage is conferred by a transgene expression <u>in association with</u> long-lived transduced cells such as T-lymphocytes may prove critical.

   ✓ The selective advantage conferred by transgene expression and long-lived transduced cells may be critical to the success of gene therapy.

5 ✖ <u>The results of this randomised, double-blind, placebo-controlled trial</u> demonstrated that this drug is effective for the treatment of seizures in children and adults. This is the first study to demonstrate a <u>statistically significant effect of this drug compared with a placebo</u> in patients with seizures.

   ✓ This is the first time that this drug has been shown to be effective for the treatment of seizures.

6 ✖ <u>Patient</u> compliance with medication regimens <u>is an area that is seen as being important because of the relationship between</u> health-related behaviours and the short- and long-term outcomes of disease.

   ✓ Compliance with medication regimens is an important research area because health behaviours are related to short- and long-term disease outcomes.

to imagine how you would explain what you want to say to a colleague or to family or friends who know nothing of your work. Once you have spoken your thoughts in a simple and straightforward way, it is often much easier to write them clearly. For this reason, studies that have been presented at conferences are more easily written up as papers than studies that have not had this advantage.

Say what you mean

There goes the man that writ a book that neither he nor anybody else understands.

(A student remarking on Sir Isaac Newton and his monumental book on mathematics called The Principia)

As scientists, we always need to convey a clear and precise meaning. Although we all know what we mean and can describe what we mean when questioned, writing can be more difficult. In scientific writing, it is important to select words that have a clear meaning and that are not open to different interpretations. You may know what you mean when you write *being exposed to environmental tobacco smoke and sex were important risk factors for childhood infections* but the words *gender* or *being male* would have been a better word choice than *sex*. Also reordering the phrases would help so that the sentence is *Gender and being exposed to environmental tobacco smoke were important risk factors for childhood infections.*

As shown in Box 8.4, you need to use phrases that are unambiguous. In each example, you can see how the meaning becomes clearer when the correct words are used. In the first example, diagnosis is not an event that can recur in an individual and so the term *less often diagnosed* is inappropriate. The second example suggests that a rat can be culled more than once, which is clearly impossible. The third example suggests that atopy, symptoms, and asthma increase in adults as they put on more weight rather than saying that overweight people have a higher prevalence of symptoms, as is intended.

Box 8.4 Saying what you mean

1 ✗ Dermatitis in the first year of life was <u>less often diagnosed</u> in the active intervention group.
   ✓ A diagnosis of dermatitis in the first year of life was less prevalent in the active intervention group.

2 ✗ Professor Jones has agreed that we can have access to some of his rats <u>that are culled on a regular basis</u>.
   ✓ Professor Jones will provide a regular supply of tissue from culled rats.

3 ✗ Although adults with severe obesity reported <u>increased</u> symptoms of wheeze and shortness of breath, this was not associated with <u>an increase in</u> atopy or asthma.
   ✓ Severely obese adults have a higher prevalence of wheeze and shortness of breath but do not have a higher prevalence of atopy or asthma.

4 ✗ After five days, the symptoms had <u>improved</u>.
   ✓ After five days, the symptoms had abated.

5 ✗ Not all cases of this illness occur in the presence of a family history and these sporadic cases present <u>some further difficulties</u> to the clinician.
   ✓ Sporadic cases of this illness that occur in the absence of a family history may be difficult to diagnose accurately.

6 ✗ This test has long been used as a surrogate estimate of disease severity and despite <u>being called into question</u> has remained in widespread use.
   ✓ This test has been used to measure disease severity since the early 1970s and, despite having poor prognostic value, remains in widespread use.

7 ✗ The calves are thin due to muscle hypertrophy around the lower leg, although adipose psuedohypertrophy has also been reported in rare cases and should be considered when <u>evaluating the clinical picture</u>.
   ✓ Muscle hypertrophy and, in rare cases, adipose psuedo-hypertrophy result in thin lower legs and are important clinical signs for making a diagnosis and evaluating prognosis.

8 ✗ Positive controls <u>have been a problem</u> for all units around the world.
   ✓ All research units have found it difficult to recruit positive controls.

> 9 ✖ As a comparator between cases, family history and the frequency of symptoms <u>are not well correlated with</u> clinical disease severity.
> ✓ Because family history and the frequency of symptoms are not related to disease severity, they cannot be used to identify subtypes of this disease.

In examples 4 to 8 in Box 8.4, the underlined words are open to interpretation and are replaced with more precise and unambiguous terms. In example 9, the word *correlated* is not a good verb to use. The word *correlate* has a specific statistical meaning and should only be used in this context. The word should not be used in a general sense to suggest that two factors are related in some way.

Word order

For your born writer, nothing is so healing as the realization that he has come upon the right word.

Catherine Brinker Bowen
(www.bartelby.com)

The correct sequencing of words within a sentence is of paramount importance. If you don't put your words in the correct order, your messages will not flow logically and your sentence will not make sense at first read. The following classified advertisement which appeared in a local newspaper is a good example of incorrect word order: *Stock horse stallions standing at stud: Reverlee and Freckles Oak. Foals can be viewed by the above stallions.*

Readers should not have to reorganise words to decipher the correct meaning. Neither should readers have to get to the end of a sentence to find out what they needed to know at the beginning. Box 8.5 shows examples of sentences that read more clearly when the words are reordered. In the first example, the word *asthma* is used incorrectly as an adjective and, because the increase in prevalence is the topic of the sentence, this phrase is better placed at the beginning. This sentence benefits from making the sentence into one main clause and from removing some of the prepositions.

In the second example, the sentence works better when the word *less* is used correctly to describe the word *prone* rather than the error. In the third example, the essential phrase, *In indigenous people who attended the emergency department*, is better placed at the beginning of the sentence so that you don't have to read all the way to the end of the sentence to discover to which group the results apply.

In the fourth example, the transition word *however* is misplaced within the sentence. Transition words or conjunctions do their job in maintaining flow better if they are used at the beginning of a sentence rather than interrupting the subject–verb–object flow. Also, the word *current* is better used as an adjective to further describe the type of information than as the adverb *currently* to describe the verb.

Box 8.5 The order of words is important

1 ✖ Although it is well recognised that asthma prevalence is increasing, this has occurred only in children and not in adults.
  ✓ An increase in the prevalence of asthma has been documented in children but not in adults.

2 ✖ Because objective measurements are prone to less observer error and reporting bias, they are preferred for use as primary outcome measures.
  ✓ Because objective measurements are less prone to observer error and reporting bias, they are preferred for use as primary outcome measures.

3 ✖ The prevalence of atopy to rye grass pollen was 24% in indigenous people who attended the emergency department.
  ✓ In indigenous people who attended the emergency department, the prevalence of atopy to rye grass pollen was 24%.

4 ✖ There is, however, currently no information about the burden of cerebral palsy in NSW.
  ✓ However, there is no current information about the burden of cerebral palsy in NSW.

The order in which you present the information in each sentence also depends on the context in which you are writing and the audience you are writing for. Sentences that work best are those in which the subject of the sentence is the main topic of your study. In this way, you provide the most important information at the beginning of the sentence and you set the context correctly. For example, you may have conducted a cross-sectional study in which you measured the risk of children developing gastrointestinal infections and investigated whether this was associated with breastfeeding. Box 8.6 shows how you might change the topic of your sentence according to whether you are reporting your study for a gastrointestinal journal, a paediatric journal, or an epidemiological journal. The data may be from the same study but your choice of word order is important for delivering a clear message to your audience.

Box 8.6 Changing the order in your topic sentences

Gastrointestinal context	Gastrointestinal infections were less common in infants who were breastfed.
Infant feeding context	Breastfeeding significantly reduced the incidence of gastrointestinal infections in infancy.
Epidemiological context	There was a lower incidence of gastrointestinal infections in breastfed infants.

Rearranging words can be just as much fun as rearranging numbers. One fun thing to do with numbers is to arrange 1 to 9 in a magic square so that the rows, columns and diagonals all have the sum of 15. Try it – it doesn't take long (the answer is at the end of this chapter). This magic square is called the *Lo Shu*.[8] If arranging numbers can be fun and satisfying, so can rearranging your words.

Creating flow

Writing, when properly managed, ... is but a different name for conversation.

Laurence Sterne (1713–1768)

Clarity depends on a smooth flow of ideas and a smooth transition between sentences and between paragraphs. In addition to making your paragraphs look nice, it is important to create flow because this allows the mind to travel along a path to instant understanding. Fellow researchers and clinicians need to be able to read your text once and understand what it means without their thoughts being left in temporary suspension at unexpected junctions. No reader wants to endure endless "stop and think" pauses to decipher how an idea in one sentence links to the ideas in the next. Writing that flows and is easy on the mind will always be appreciated.

There are two main methods for maintaining a flow of ideas from one sentence to the next. One method is to use conjunctions or transition words to link sentences. Classical transition words, such as *although, therefore, however, for example,* etc., are useful for joining things together. Nevertheless, you cannot keep using transition words throughout a paragraph. Box 8.7 shows a paragraph in which a transition word is used to begin each sentence. The messages of the paragraph are reasonably clear but the overload of transition words reduces rather than aids readability. Although transition words work occasionally, other skills are also needed to create flow.

Box 8.7 Using transition words to begin sentences

In addition, it is widely recognised that most cases of child sexual abuse are not reported to authorities. Therefore, prevalence rates that include reported and unreported cases more accurately describe the extent of the problem of child sexual assaults in communities. However, cases are difficult to ascertain through retrospective population studies. For example, there is an inverse association between study response rates and the estimated prevalence of child sexual abuse.

Another method to create flow between sentences is to link the beginning (or subject) of the sentence to the end (or object) of the previous sentence. Linking subjects to objects between sentences helps to maintain ideas in the reader's mind because it avoids any abrupt change of thoughts when a full stop is reached.

The examples in Box 8.8 show that by simply reordering the words and creating an *object-to-subject* flow between sentences, the ideas are carried forwards and do not jar the mind. In examples 1–3, the second sentence is simply reordered. Even if the linking word can't be moved to the very beginning of the second sentence, moving it as close as possible still helps. In example 4, the reference to *prevalence* is moved closer to the beginning of the second sentence and the new concept, *incidence*, is moved to the end, clarifying the message.

Box 8.8 Creating flow between sentences

1 ✖ Obesity is a key risk factor for cardiovascular disease. In Australia, over 50% of adults are overweight or obese.

✓ In Australia, over 50% of adults are overweight or obese. Being overweight is a significant risk factor for the development of cardiovascular disease.

2 ✖ We conducted a study of children of whom 10% had diabetes. We found a higher incidence of obesity in children with diabetes.

✓ We conducted a study of children of whom 10% had diabetes. Children with diabetes have a higher incidence of obesity.

3 ✖ We found that 43% of parents smoked. Children were at a higher risk of having respiratory infections if their parents smoked.

✓ We found that 43% of parents smoked. Children with a parent who smokes are at higher risk of having respiratory infections.

4 ✖ Prevalence is calculated from the total number of cases of disease in a population at a specified time. Unlike the incidence rate, the number of remissions and deaths that occur influences the prevalence rate.

✓ Prevalence is the proportion of a population with a disease at a specified time. The number of remissions and deaths influences prevalence rates but not incidence rates.

In addition to creating continuity by using good transitions, repeating key terms throughout a paragraph can also help to maintain thought processes. However, it is a good idea to avoid using the same word twice in one sentence because this becomes boring. Also, repeating a word in a sentence usually signals a construction problem because it does not make sense for the same word to be both the subject and the object of a sentence. The examples in Box 8.9 show how sentences become neater and more interesting when the words are reorganised and the repeated term is removed.

Box 8.9 Avoiding repetitions

1　✖ We need reliable screening procedures for <u>identifying</u> the signs and symptoms to <u>identify</u> children who are at greatest risk.
　✓ We need reliable screening tools to identify children who are at greatest risk.

2　✖ No adequate <u>clinical</u> measures for quantifying back abnormalities in the <u>clinical</u> setting are currently available.
　✓ There are no adequate methods for quantifying back abnormalities in clinical settings.

3　✖ The results of this study suggest that <u>control of neonatal infections</u> is possible through good <u>infection control</u> practices.
　✓ The results of this study suggest that neonatal infections are being reduced by current infection control practices.

Tight writing

Cutting dross allows your information to shine more clearly. In the early 1900s, Professor William Strunk used to tell his students: "Omit needless words, omit needless words, omit needless words." (Once should have been enough, but he was keen.)

Martin Cutts[9]

Tight writing is the art of achieving brevity by using short, concise sentences. Given that every book or article on writing recommends this style as a matter of course, it is surprising that so few writers aspire to this ideal. Readers love sentences and paragraphs that have a minimum number of words and that only include the information that they really need.

You must write tightly if you want to please your readers. Readers are busy people who want to be able to understand your paper quickly and do not want to spend time sorting out meanings from meandering text. Tight writing is a simple process. All you have to do is put your thoughts down in a sentence, then be your own best critic and see how many words you can leave out. Finally, when you have a series of short, concise sentences, you need to arrange them in a logical order and join them up to create flow. In doing this, you suddenly have a neat way to tell your story. This is a skill that is certainly worth perfecting if you would like to publish productively. If you follow this formula, you will automatically please your readers, reviewers, and publishers. In doing this, you will also earn yourself respect as a "good writer", which is a reputation worth striving for. Box 8.10 shows how removing long or redundant phrases improves readability.

Box 8.10 Removing long or redundant phrases

1 ✖ Sexual assault <u>against a child presents a significant problem to society and there is much evidence that sexual assault</u> impacts negatively on the psychosocial development of children.
   ✓ Sexual assault has a negative impact on the psychosocial development of children.

2 ✖ <u>It may be expected that</u> the prevalence of <u>relatively</u> mild asthma could be underestimated.
   ✓ The prevalence of mild asthma could have been underestimated.

3 ✖ The severity of this disease <u>has been demonstrated to be associated</u> with age.
   ✓ The severity of this disease increases with age.

If you are finding it hard to write tightly, it is a good idea to put your draft away for some time and then revisit it when you can be more objective. When you are ready to revise it, begin with a plan to keep your sentences as precise as possible. Inspect your long sentences and decide whether they are overburdened with adjectives, adverbs, prepositions, and pronouns. However, if you cut a sentence into two, ensure that each short sentence stands alone in that its meaning is clear even when it is isolated from its neighbours or from the remainder of the paragraph.

If you are having problems in trying to shorten your sentences, a good trick is to first identify the main "subject–verb–object" section and then prune away at the remainder. After you have done this, inspect your verb construction and ask yourself if it could be shorter. For example, constructions such as *has been shown to be* can often be replaced by *is* if the evidence is definitive or *may be* if the evidence is less certain. When the extraneous words and repetitions are removed, the readability of the sentence suddenly improves.

In shortening sentences, do not go to extremes. You must resist deleting necessary details simply to cut words. If you oversimplify a sentence so that the true meaning is lost, you will achieve brevity at the expense of clarity. For example, it is better to say *We are planning to conduct a study of preventive health services for children with Down syndrome* than to say *We are doing a study of preventive health services for children with Down syndrome*. The latter is shorter but suggests that you are working on it at this present moment whereas the first sentence is factually correct.

Box 8.11 shows how reducing words, simplifying messages, and omitting needless phrases can achieve brevity and clarity and improve the readability of both the title and the text. The mean number of words per sentence is only reduced from 29·6 with a range of 19–37 words in the original version to 29·0 with a range of 22–35 words in the revised version. However, the total word count has been reduced from 205 to 114 (a 46% reduction) and the number of sentences from 7 to 4 (a 44% reduction). It all depends on what you want to achieve. Tight writing creates text that is easy and enjoyable for your audience to read and displays a high regard for both your peers and reviewers, who are almost always busy people.

Box 8.11 Example of reducing words to achieve brevity and clarity

✖ Original version

Development of a composite, criterion-based, observational, clinical rating system for the quantification of back posture

There are a number of existing methods for assessing back posture in the clinical setting but all have significant limitations. Many measures have been criticised for poor reliability, and few have been subjected to adequate validation, furthermore most extant measures are based on quantification of a single plane or segment. While such measures are widely used, they cannot describe the complexity of back function, and there is a consensus in the literature that there is not an adequate, quantitative method for assessing back posture in routine clinical practice. The 1997 report of the Research Council of the American Physical Therapy Society rated development of such outcome measures as the third most important research area out of 40 separate categories. This study represents the second of six stages in constructing such a clinically applicable tool, the Back Posture Rating (BPR). Emphasis has been placed on clinical measures that could be conducted easily, are time-efficient, do not require costly technology, are readily understandable to the clinician, and yield quantitative data at a minimum of ordinal level. The combination of measures comprising the BPR is also sensitive to posture in all of the three body planes and can provide separable information on the high, mid, and lower segments.

✓ Revised version

Clinical assessment of back posture

Methods for quantifying back problems have lacked reliability, have not been validated and, because they are based on a single plane or segment, do not take account of the complex nature of back function. As a result, the American Physical Therapy Society rated the development of a back function measurement as its third most important research goal. The aim of conducting this study was to test the reliability of a new Back Posture Rating (BPR) that is practical to administer in a clinic setting. Because this rating measures movement in all three planes, it is a sensitive measure of back posture and can provide separate information about the high, mid and lower back segments.

In tight writing you only say things once. The practice of saying something twice in one sentence is known as tautology and is described in the *Oxford English Dictionary* as "a fault of style". For example, there is no need to say that you studied *the subsequent development of infection*. Since development can only be subsequent, the word *subsequent* is unnecessary. Also, do not describe something as being *equally as important* since the word *equally* is redundant. Similarly, in the sentence, *There is no need to repeat the tests again*, the word *repeat* can be replaced by *conduct*, or the word *again* can be deleted. It is amazing how often scientists use extraneous words, and how much clearer their writing would be if they didn't.

Box 8.12 shows some examples of sentences that include unnecessary words. In the first example, cross-sectional studies are large random population studies by definition, so only one of the two phrases is needed. The sentence also benefits from being rearranged so that the descriptor *obese* is not separated from its noun *adults*.

In the second example, the word *very* is not needed because there are no degrees of inaccuracy. Moreover, the sentence is better written with the topic, which is the measurement of diet, as the subject. In the third example, time can only be a period so *a considerable period of* is redundant. It always pays to be precise in scientific writing so the more specific phrase *for 12 years* is even better. In the fourth and fifth examples, the tautologies can simply be removed.

Box 8.12 Examples of tautologies

1 ✗ In adults, <u>cross-sectional studies in large random population samples</u> have shown a higher prevalence of asthma among obese subjects.
  ✓ Evidence from <u>cross-sectional population studies</u> suggests that the prevalence of asthma is higher in adults who are obese.

2 ✗ This questionnaire is likely to produce <u>very inaccurate</u> estimates of dietary intake.
  ✓ Most dietary measurements <u>will be inaccurate</u> if this questionnaire is used.

3 ✗ We studied our subjects over a <u>considerable period of time</u>.
  ✓ We continued to follow our participants <u>for 12 years</u>.

4 ✗ When designing a study, the <u>primary key issue</u> is to articulate the aims.
  ✓ When designing a study, the <u>key issue</u> is to articulate the aims.

5 ✗ <u>To date, no recent information</u> is available about children who present to hospital with this condition.
  ✓ <u>No information</u> is available about children who present to hospital with this condition.

Chopping up snakes

The writer's aim should be to be understood at first reading. It is your responsibility to be clear – not your reader's to unscramble your muddled message.

Elizabeth Murphy[3]

Short sentences are the crux of good scientific writing. Sentences with few words convey their meaning clearly at the first reading. If you are prone to writing long, snake-like sentences you will have to learn to chop them up.[10]

Instead of making a single point, long sentences usually try and convey too much information in one go. Long sentences quickly exhaust thinking capacity and are hard work to read. Snakes overload the reader who has to search for the main message while trying to remember and place all of the subtopics and asides. If a sentence has too many phrases and clauses, readers will not be able to maintain all the ideas until they reach the full stop. Long sentences may occasionally be needed but they should be the exception rather than the rule.

It's hard to generalise how long is too long. One rule of thumb is that sentences that stretch to more than two printed lines and/or more than 30 words are too long. Sentences longer than this suddenly become tedious and difficult to read whereas sentences with less than 20 words are usually very readable. Simply by chopping up the snakes, you make your paragraphs more digestible. Cut long sentences into little ones, shorten verbs, delete unnecessary clauses, or put points in a list. It doesn't matter how you achieve shortness, but for clear writing it is important that you do.

Box 8.13 shows that by removing unnecessary words and by including a full stop in the middle of the sentences and starting again, you give your readers a breather to digest the latest point

---

Box 8.13 Chopping up snakes

- ✖ We did not collect any precise information about infections but we found that having bronchitis before the age of two was a strong, independent risk factor for both wheeze and diagnosed asthma in indigenous children although it is possible that indigenous children who had bronchitis in early life were more likely to be diagnosed with asthma than non-indigenous children who had bronchitis.

- ✓ We did not collect objective information about infections but we found that bronchitis before the age of two was a strong risk factor for wheeze and diagnosed asthma in indigenous children. Although we have no evidence, it is possible that indigenous children who have bronchitis in early life are more likely to be diagnosed with asthma.

and prepare themselves for the next. The long snaky sentence of 63 words can easily be cut into two sentences, one of 32 words and one of 25 words (total 57 words).

Parallel structures

To be easy to read, your text has to be clear and say what you mean in a simple and straightforward way. It has been said that clear text is easy to read but hard to write.

JS Lilleyman[11]

By using the same sequences of word clusters both within and between sentences, you create "parallel sentence structures". Parallel structures improve readability by creating a smooth, organised flow of thought. By establishing repetitive patterns, you introduce good structure to your writing because you present your ideas in a consistent way.

Sentences that have an inconsistent, or non-parallel, structure inhibit thought patterns. By giving too many ideas that are presented in different word orders from one another, non-parallel sentences can become brain-teasers. Box 8.14 shows how to make sentences parallel simply by changing the grammatical construction.

Box 8.14 Examples of parallel sentences

1. ✘ To study mechanisms and investigate risk factors will provide useful information.
   ✓ Studying mechanisms and investigating risk factors will provide useful information.
   ✓ To study mechanisms and to investigate risk factors will provide useful information.

2. ✘ Dr Smith's idea is brilliant, original, and will work.
   ✓ Dr Smith's idea is brilliant, is original, and will work.
   ✓ Dr Smith's idea is brilliant, original, and practical.

In the first example, different forms of the two verbs (to study and to investigate) are used. By standardising the verb form, the sentence becomes parallel. In the second example, the list needs to be standardised. You can write a list in which each item has a verb or you can write a list in which no items have a verb, but the list must be consistent.

Box 8.15 shows some examples of non-parallel sentences with suggestions about how to amend them. The first example is difficult to understand because the two different methods of describing the data from men and women are inconsistent. By simply making *overweight* the object of the sentence rather than an adjective in the first clause and by standardising the way in which results from the two studies are described, the message becomes much easier to comprehend.

In the second example, there are four items in the list. The first two and the final item are each reported in a consistent "subject–verb–object way." However, the third item has the verb at the end in a subject (*follow up*)–object (*cohort*)–verb (*are undertaken*) structure that is non-parallel to the other items. This confuses readers who expect to be able to process the words in the same order in each clause. The sentence becomes clearer when the third item becomes parallel by moving the verb to the centre and when two items with the same subject (*follow up assessments*) are merged. Finally, the phrase *during the study* is redundant and can be omitted. The sentence is reduced by only four words but the parallelism and therefore the flow and the readability are improved significantly.

Similarly, in the third example, the sentence becomes clearer when the percentage is placed before the verb in both clauses rather than at the beginning of one clause and end of the next. If you are comparing two groups, always make one group the comparison group as shown in the fourth example. In the corrected sentence, indigenous children are the group of interest, and non-indigenous children, in the context of the study, are the control group. This avoids confusion in trying to understand which illnesses were more or less prevalent in which group.

Parallelism can also be achieved between sentences by making them match one another in construction. If you are comparing data from two groups, then always cite the groups in the same order. For example, if you are comparing the prevalence of a disease in children and adults then always cite the data for children before the data for adults throughout your paper.

Box 8.15 Making sentence structures parallel

1 ✖ One study found that only 15% of overweight men and 5% of overweight women considered their weight to be acceptable and the other study found that 25% of men and 45% of women of acceptable weight considered themselves to be overweight.
✓ In one study, 15% of men and 5% of women who were overweight considered their weight acceptable whilst in another study, 25% of men and 45% of women with acceptable weight considered themselves overweight.

2 ✖ Longitudinal studies are most useful if the cohort is selected as a random sample of the general population, if follow up continues from childhood to adulthood, and if several follow up assessments of the cohort are undertaken during the study and if the outcomes include objective measurements.
✓ Longitudinal studies are most useful if the cohort is selected as a random sample of the general population, if follow up assessments continue from childhood to adulthood and are conducted at regular intervals, and if the outcomes include objective measurements.

3 ✖ Disability was reported by 58% of the respondents as interfering with their professional capacity and to be restricting leisure activities in 70% of the group.
✓ In this study, 58% of participants reported that their disability interfered with their professional capacity and 70% reported that their disability restricted their leisure activities.

4 ✖ The prevalence of asthma was higher in non-indigenous children but the prevalence of infections was higher in indigenous children.
✓ The prevalence of asthma was lower but the prevalence of infections was higher in indigenous children.

Style matters

Proper words in proper places make the true definition of a style.

Jonathan Swift, (1667–1745, in *Letter to a young clergyman*)

Table 8.1 Style table for scientific writing

Tip	Action
Write the topic sentence	✓ Begin each paragraph with a topic sentence and use the main subject of the paper as the subject of the sentence
Draft the remainder of the paragraph	✓ Follow the topic sentence with supporting sentences
Put the sentences in the correct order	✓ Check for logic in the order in which you present ideas
Eliminate fog	✓ Simplify your thoughts and your sentences ✓ Avoid jargon and acronyms ✓ Use everyday words
Say what you mean	✓ Inspect word orders and word meanings
Ensure flow between sentences	✓ Link end of one sentence to beginning of next or use transition words
Write tight	✓ Delete all non-essential words, phrases, and clauses
Chop up the snakes	✓ Use short sentences of about 20–30 words
Check for non-parallelism	✓ Maintain consistent viewpoints and orders within and between sentences
Think of your audience	✓ Imagine you are explaining your work to a fellow researcher
Make your paper look attractive	✓ Chop up walls of text and keep changes of topic visual (new paragraph) and verbal (new topic sentence)

In summary, a few simple writing rules can help you to achieve clarity and brevity in your writing. The tips that have been discussed in this chapter are summarised in Table 8.1. By following a few simple rules, you can improve your writing style. As a result, your work will be more publishable and you will receive greater respect from your colleagues.

Solution to magic square

The answer to the magic square puzzle is as follows:

4	9	2
3	5	7
8	1	6

Acknowledgements

The Hitchcock, Sterne and Swift qutoes have been produced with permission from *Collins Concise Dictionary of Quotations, 3rd edn*. London: Harper Collins, 1998 (p 160, 307, 311 respectively). The student remarking on Sir Isaac Newton quote has been produced with permission from Horvitz, LA ed. *The Quotable Scientist*. New York: McGraw-Hill Companies, 2000 (p 115). King quotes have been reprinted with the permission of Scribner, a Division of Simon & Schuster, Inc., from *On Writing: A Memoir of the Craft* by Stephen King. Copyright © by Stephen King. All other referenced quotes have been produced with permission.

Websites

1 Bartelby Online Books
http://www.bartelby.com
Access to online books such as the *American Heritage® dictionary, American Heritage® book of English usage, Roget's thesaurus, Strunk's elements of style, Gray's anatomy*, etc.

2 Modern Language Association (MLA) of America
http://www.mla.org
http://www.mla.org/main_stl.htm#sources
Information about the MLA style manual which documents the style recommended by the Modern Language Association for preparing scholarly manuscripts and student research papers. Concerns itself with the mechanics of writing, such as punctuation, quotation, and documentation of sources. Also includes guidelines for citing sources from the World Wide Web

3 Plain English Campaign
http://www.plainenglish.co.uk
Guides to writing medical information, letters, reports, alternative words, etc. for writing in plain English

4 The Writing Program, University of Pennsylvania
http://www.sas.upenn.edu/writing/services/docs.html

Access to online reference texts and resources including *Grammar Style and Notes* by Jack Lynch, *Strunk's Elements of Style*, *Oxford English Dictionary*, *Webster's Dictionary*, *Roget's Thesaurus*, citation styles, etc.

5 Yahoo
http://dir.yahoo.com/Social_Science/Linguistics_and_
Human_Languages/Languages/Specific_Languages/
English/Grammar_Usage_and_Style/
Access to resources for grammar, English usage and style, including books and rules of grammar, common errors, and tips to improve your writing

References

1 Zeiger M. *Essentials of writing biomedical research papers*. Maidenhead: McGraw-Hill, 1991; p 3.
2 Australian Government Publishing Service. *Spot on*. Correspondence and report writing with guidelines in plain English. Canberra: AGPS, 1996; p 2.
3 Murphy E. *Effective writing*. : Longman Cheshire Pty Ltd, 1989; pp 1, 5.
4 Zeiger M. Paragraph structure. *In Essentials of writing biomedical research papers*. Maidenhead: McGraw-Hill, 1991.
5 Eisenhut M, Algawi B, Wreghitt T, *et al*. Fatal coxsackie A9 virus infection during an outbreak in a neonatal unit. *J Infection* 2000;**40**:297–8.
6 Peat JK, Tovey ER, Toelle BG, *et al*. House-dust mite allergens: a major risk factor for childhood asthma in Australia. *Am J Respir Crit Care Med* 1996;**153**:141–6.
7 King S. *On writing*. London: Scribner, 2000; p 117.
8 Spencer A. *Book of numbers*. London: Penguin Books, 2000.
9 Cutts M. *The plain English guide*. Oxford: Oxford University Press, 1996; p 40.
10 Cutts M. Writing shorter sentences … or chopping up snakes. In: *The plain English guide*. Oxford: Oxford University Press, 1995.
11 Lilleyman JS. How to write a scientific paper – a rough guide to getting published. *Arch Dis Child* 1995;**72**:268–70.

9: Grammar

*So much of writing is about sitting down and doing it
every day, and so much of it is about getting into the
custom of taking in everything that comes along, seeing
it all as grist for the mill.*

Anne Lamott[1]

The objectives of this chapter are to understand how to:

- write grammatically correct sentences
- know what sentence constructions you need to use and why
- categorise words and know why they are there
- avoid common grammatical mistakes
- write in perfect English

A sentence is a group of words that convey a complete
thought. To do this clearly, sentences need to conform to
established rules about organising words, which is where
grammar comes in. For some of us, this word brings back
memories of incomprehensible rules that were part of our
school's mantra. For others, grammar is a mystery because the
rules never made it on to our school curriculum. If you didn't
learn grammar at school or if you have forgotten the grammar
that you did learn, it's a good idea to brush up on some of the
elementary terms and rules.

Most of us know when sentences read well and when they
don't. Grammar is about knowing why something reads badly
and knowing how to fix it. It is impossible to write well without
using words correctly. In this chapter, we demystify some of the
terms and rules of grammar to help you find simple and correct
ways of grouping words into sentences. We also explain the
names of each part of a sentence and show you into which
categories the words used in Box 3.2 (Chapter 3) fall.

Nouns

> *Don't be intimidated. Grammar books aren't as forbidding and textbooky as they used to be, and not all of them bristle with technical terms. You don't need to know the heavy terminology anyway. You can be a good driver even if you can't name all the parts of a car.*
>
> Patricia O'Conner[2]

Nouns are words that describe something concrete such as a person or an object. This is not surprising since the word "noun" is Latin for "name". The subjects and objects of sentences are nouns or groups of words that function as a noun.

Examples of nouns that come to mind are those that describe people, such as *student, participant, researcher,* or *writer*, and nouns that describe objects, such as *computer, ruler, questionnaire,* or *mass spectrometer*. There are also nouns that describe places, such as *laboratory, clinic,* and *home*, and nouns that describe intangibles, such as *health, time,* and *temperature*. Proper nouns are a special class of nouns. These nouns are the names of people or places and always begin with a capital letter, such as *London, America,* or *James*. Sometimes nouns are strung together to make noun clusters or phrases, such as *peer review, research study*, etc.

Nouns are the concrete material of our text that we glue together with verbs and pronouns and that we decorate with adjectives. Box 9.1 shows the nouns that were used in Box 3.2 in Chapter 3. In most sentences, the subjects and objects are clearly identified as a noun or noun cluster, although some sentences end in a verb such as *investigated* or an adjective such as *reliable*. The noun cluster *National Nutrition Survey*, which has two adjectives before the noun, is capitalised because it is a formal name of a study and *Australia* is capitalised because it a proper noun. Forming word clusters can be useful and efficient but should be used sparingly to avoid continuous strings of nouns making the text dense and tortuous to read.

> **Box 9.1 Use of nouns (underlined) in an introduction section**
>
> **Introduction**
>
> <u>People</u> who are overweight or obese are at increased <u>risk</u> of developing many <u>illnesses</u> including <u>hypertension</u>, cardiovascular <u>disease</u> and non-insulin dependent <u>diabetes</u>. However, many <u>adults</u> continue to be overweight. In 1995, <u>results</u> from the National Nutrition <u>Survey</u> in <u>Australia</u> suggested that 63% of <u>men</u> and 47% of <u>women</u> were either overweight or obese.
>
> Despite the <u>impact</u> of excess body <u>weight</u> on <u>health</u>, <u>self-perception</u> of body <u>mass</u> in the general <u>population</u> has not been properly investigated. The only <u>information</u> comes from small, unrepresentative <u>samples</u> of <u>women</u>, particularly younger <u>women</u>, or from national <u>studies</u> in which self-reported <u>weights</u> may be unreliable. Until reliable <u>information</u> of <u>self-perceptions</u> of body <u>mass</u> is collected, it is difficult to design effective weight loss intervention <u>strategies</u>.
>
> In 1998, we conducted a large cross-sectional <u>survey</u> of <u>adults</u> in which we accurately measured <u>height</u> and <u>weight</u>. In this <u>paper</u>, we report <u>information</u> about adults' <u>perceptions</u> of their own body <u>mass</u>.

The nouns from Box 9.1 can be classified into their various types as shown in Table 9.1. Nouns that describe people, objects, or places are usually very easily identified because they describe something concrete. However, nouns that describe intangibles are harder to identify because they describe something that can't be seen or touched.

Table 9.1 Classifying the nouns shown in Box 9.1.

Type of noun	Nouns used
Describes people	people, adults, men, women
Describes objects	factors, results, survey, information, samples, studies, strategies, survey, paper
Describes a place	Australia
Describes intangibles	risk, illnesses, impact, hypertension, disease, diabetes, impact, weight, health, self-perception, mass, height, perceptions

If you are having trouble sorting out nouns from some verb forms, try putting *a* or *the* before the word. If it sounds right, the word is almost certainly a noun. If in doubt, consult your dictionary.

Sneaky plurals

> *Some years ago, when the heir to the throne of England was a child, I noticed a headline in* The Times *about* Bonnie Prince Charlie: *"Charles' tonsils out". Immediately Rule 1 leapt to mind: "Form the possessive singular of nouns by adding's. Follow this rule whatever the final consonant." Thus, write "Charles's friend".*
>
> William Strunk Jr[3]

When nouns are used in a plural form, the general convention is to add an "s" to the end of the word. Thus, the plural of the singular noun *interval* is *intervals*. When the singular noun is used, it is always matched with a singular verb as in *The interval is* ... and, when the plural noun is used, it is matched with a plural verb as in *The intervals are*.

This convention of adding an "s" to form a plural works well for most words except words of Latin or Greek origin. For example, *formulae* is the plural of *formula* and *criteria* is the plural of *criterion*. Some obscure plurals to be on the look out for are those such as *media,* which is the plural of *medium,* and *data* which is the plural of the rarely used Latin word *datum*. In matching the word *data* with a verb, you must never write *the data is* but rather be grammatically correct and write *the data are*. However, if you are writing about a data bank, the noun *bank* is singular and so you write *the data bank is stored here*.

Some nouns such as the words *police* and *children* are plural nouns in their own right that refer to a collection of people. To be grammatically correct, these collective nouns require a plural verb so we write *the children are*. However, to make things complicated, some collective nouns take a singular verb, such as *the team has* or *the government is*. When writing any sentence it is important that you identify the subject and the verb and ensure that they match in terms of both being singular or both being plural. If you are unsure, try putting the indefinite article *a* before the noun. If this makes sense, the word is singular since *a* means *one of* and it then needs a singular verb. Some examples of sneaky plurals are shown in Box 9.2.

Box 9.2 Examples of sneaky plurals

1 ✖ Data <u>is</u> presented as means with their 95% confidence intervals
   ✓ Data are presented as means with their 95% confidence intervals

2 ✖ A random sample of sixty homes <u>were</u> selected to have dust collected
   ✓ A random sample of sixty homes was selected to have dust collected
   ✓ Dust was collected from a random sample of 60 homes

3 ✖ When you decide where to publish your paper, you should obtain the list of instructions to authors and read <u>them</u> carefully
   ✓ When you decide where to publish your paper, you should obtain the list of instructions to authors and read it carefully

---

In example 1, the correct verb to use with the plural noun *data* is *are* and not *is* as discussed above. In the second example, the verb *were* belongs to the noun *sample* and should be similarly singular. This sentence is better when written in a more direct way with the word *dust* at the beginning of the sentence as the subject, and where it was collected from (*a random sample of 60 homes*) at the end as the object. In the third example, the pronoun *them* is referring to *the list* and not to *instructions* and should also be similarly singular.

Notes on nouns

Do not be tempted to use some nouns as verbs or adjectives. For example, the word *impact* is a noun. It is better to write that *your talk had an impact on the audience* rather than *your talk impacted on the audience.*

Some mistakes arise from incorrectly using a noun as an adjective. For example, it is not a good idea to write *in the Colorado study* but rather to write *in the study undertaken in Colorado* or *in the American study*. The difference is that *American* is an adjective whereas *Colorado* is a proper noun that should not be used as an adjective.

Similarly, the word *correlation* is a noun. Therefore, you cannot write *This correlation study indicated a significant relation between drug concentration and markers of renal function* in which *correlation* is used as an adjective. Moreover, the different types of research studies are described in Chapter 3 and a *correlation study* is not one of them. To avoid ambiguity, only use the word *correlation* when you are reporting results obtained by using a correlation coefficient.

In describing ethnic groups, it is especially important not to use adjectives in place of a noun. For example, we should always write about *Aborigines*. This word is a plural noun and is the correct term to describe indigenous people. It is important never to use the term *Aboriginals* because *Aboriginal* is an adjective that does not have or need a plural form.

Finally, remember that the word *relation* is the correct word to use to describe what one thing has to do with another as in *We examined the relation between height and weight*. The word *relationship* is only used to describe kinship or other bonds between people.

Adjectives

> *You don't see something until you have the right metaphor to let you perceive it.*
>
> Robert Stetson Shaw (physicist)

Adjectives are words that are used to describe, or embellish, nouns. It is usually a simple matter to identify the adjectives in a sentence. For example, in the phrase *a random sample*, the word *random* is an adjective that describes the type of sample that was recruited. In fact the words *a* and *the* are also adjectives in a strict sense but generally go by their titles of indefinite and definite article respectively. The word *a* is called an "indefinite article" because, like its companion *an*, it refers to an item that has not already been specifically mentioned. On the other hand, the word *the* is called the "definite article" because it refers to a particular item.

When two or more adjectives are used in a list, they are separated by a comma as in *small, unrepresentative samples* and in *large, cross-sectional survey*. However, when adjectives are joined with a noun to form a noun cluster, as in *non-insulin dependent diabetes* or *effective weight loss intervention strategies* no comma is needed. In some sentences, the adjective almost acts like a noun when it is the object of the sentence. For example, in the phrase *self-reported weights may be unreliable*, the word *unreliable* is an adjective that describes *self-reported weights* but it acts as the object of the sentence.

Box 9.3 shows the adjectives that were used, in some cases as noun clusters, in Box 3.2 in Chapter 3. In this text, many of the nouns are qualified by adjectives. Although sentences can largely stand alone without adjectives, adjectives are needed to convey a precise rather than a general meaning.

Box 9.3 Use of adjectives (underlined) in an introduction section

People who are <u>overweight</u> or <u>obese</u> are at <u>increased</u> risk of developing <u>many</u> illnesses including hypertension, <u>cardiovascular</u> disease and <u>non-insulin dependent</u> diabetes. However, <u>many</u> adults continue to be <u>overweight</u>. In 1995, results from the <u>National Nutrition</u> Survey in Australia suggested that 63% of men and 47% of women were either <u>overweight</u> or <u>obese</u>.

Despite the impact of <u>excess body</u> weight on health, self-perception of <u>body</u> mass in the <u>general</u> population has not been properly investigated. The <u>only</u> information comes from <u>small, unrepresentative</u> samples of women, particularly <u>younger</u> women, or from <u>national</u> studies in which <u>self-reported</u> weights may be <u>unreliable</u>. Until <u>reliable</u> information of self-perceptions of <u>body</u> mass is collected, it is <u>difficult</u> to design <u>effective weight loss intervention</u> strategies.

In 1998, we conducted a <u>large, cross-sectional</u> survey of adults in which we accurately measured height and weight. In this paper, we report information about <u>adults'</u> perceptions of their <u>own body</u> mass.

Notes on adjectives

When using adjectives they need to be placed correctly to achieve a specific meaning. For example, in the sentence *I was the only one who could use the cell sorter*, the word *only* is used as an adjective to qualify the noun *one*. However, in the sentence *I was the one who could only use the cell sorter*, the word *only* is used as an adverb to qualify the verb *use*. By moving the word *only*, the sentence takes on a very different meaning.

Also remember that every study is *unique* in that no two studies are ever identical so the adjective *unique* should not be used as a descriptor of a scientific study. In addition, *unique* coupled with an adverb such as *very unique* should definitely be avoided because there are no degrees of uniqueness. No matter which granting body you are trying to sell your study to, never be tempted to write anything along the lines of *This is a truly unique cohort with a long follow up and objective outcomes*.

Verbs

> *Here's to the verb! It works harder than any other part of the sentence. The verb is the word that gets things done. Without a verb, there's nothing happening and you don't really need a sentence at all.*
>
> Patricia O'Conner[2]

Verbs are "doing words" that form the heart of a sentence. The *Oxford English Dictionary* describes verbs as "a part of speech that predicates or asserts an action" although a more spirited description of a verb is a word "that kick starts a sentence".[4] Verbs are easily recognised because they describe an action or a thought. When you put the word *to* in front of a verb, you create what is known as the infinitive form. For

Table 9.2 Types of verbs.

Verb type	Verb	Examples
Primary verbs	write	I write journal articles
	writes	He writes journal articles
	writing	He is writing a journal article
	wrote	He wrote a journal article
	written	A journal article is being written
Primary auxiliary verbs	am	I am writing a journal article
	have	I have written a journal article
	do	I do want to write a journal article
Secondary auxiliary verbs	can, could	I could write a journal article
	may, might, must	I may write a journal article
	shall, should, will, would	I shall write a journal article
Both a primary and secondary auxiliary verb	may and be	I may be writing a journal article

example, *continue* is the verb in the sentence *The study has not been continued* and is recognised by its infinitive form *to continue*. If you can create an infinitive form with a word, it is certainly a verb.

Verbs take a huge variety of forms. Primary verbs are verbs that can be used alone. The form of the primary verb is usually related to whether the action was in the past, is in the present, or will be in the future such as in *I conducted a study*, *I am conducting a study* or *I will conduct a study*. In these three verb phrases the primary verb is *to conduct*. However, the word *conduct* is used in conjunction with the auxiliary verbs *am* or *will* to convey a sense of time. Some examples of primary, primary auxiliary, and secondary auxiliary verbs are shown in Table 9.2.

For writers who really want to get into the language of verbs and grammar, a verb and its related words in a clause or a sentence is called the *predicate*. The predicate describes what the subject of the sentence did. For example, in the sentence *The study was continued for a number of years*, the underlined word group is the predicate because it tells us what happened to the study. The word or phrase that is usually a noun or an adjective and that completes the predicate and/or describes the subject is called the *complement*. In the above sentence, the phrase *for a number of years* is the complement. The complement is often a single word such as in the sentence *The man was embarrassed* where *was embarrassed* is the predicate and *embarrassed* is the complement.

To complicate matters even further, verbs can take an "active" or a "passive" form. Fortunately, computer grammar checkers often alert us if we use a passive verb form. One way to recognise the passive form without relying on computer alerts is that the verb is usually a cluster of several words and the subject often follows the verb rather than leading the sentence. For example, you can write that *People are considered to be at higher risk for having heart disease if they are obese* or that *Obesity is a risk factor for heart disease*. In the first sentence, the subject is *people* and there is a passive verb cluster *are considered to be*. However, the second sentence correctly has the subject *obesity* at the beginning and uses an active verb *is*. Use an active verb rather than a passive verb whenever possible.

The use of active verbs is a sure way to improve the readability of scientific writing. Some examples of changing long, passive verb constructions into short, active ones are shown in Box 9.4. In the first example, the verb form *has been shown to be* is certainly the passive voice and can be easily replaced with *is* or any other short form of the verb *to be*. This example also has another problem in that it is the children with attention deficit disorder who have the problems, not the disease itself. The sentence makes more sense and is better written as shown. It is important to be on the look out for faulty sentence constructions such as this. In the second example, the verbs are simply shortened without any loss of meaning.

Box 9.4 Using short verb forms

1 ✖ Attention deficit disorder <u>has been shown to be</u> associated with a wide range of problems such as poor school performance and poor peer relations

    ✓ Attention deficit disorder <u>is associated</u> with a wide range of problems such as poor school performance and poor peer relations

    ✓ Children with attention deficit disorder <u>have</u> a wide range of problems including poor school performance and poor peer relationships

2 ✖ In this study, we <u>have sought to minimise</u> the risk of recall bias by investigating preschool age children

    ✓ We <u>have minimised</u> recall bias by electing to study preschool children

---

Table 9.3 Verb tense to use throughout your paper.

Section	Verb tense	Examples
Introduction	Present or past tense for describing the evidence that exists Past tense for describing your aims or hypotheses	It is known that ... There is no evidence that ... Therefore, we investigated whether ...
Methods	Past tense throughout	Participants were recruited from ...
Results	Past tense for results Present tense to refer to tables, etc.	We found that ... Figure 1 shows that ...
Discussion	Present tense for answers to questions Present tense to discuss the literature Past tense to discuss the results	Our findings suggest that ... Evidence from cohort studies shows that ... We found that ...

The verb tense to use when you are writing a paper is well prescribed, as shown in Table 9.3. Because we are describing the aims we had when we began the study, the participants who we studied and the results that we found, these sections are limited to being written in the past tense. However, much of the introduction and discussion can be written in the present tense if you are describing the evidence that currently exists and how it relates to your hypotheses or findings.

Box 9.5 shows the verbs that were used in Box 3.2 in Chapter 3. As you can see, the majority of verbs are in the centre of their sentences and most verbs are short. In fact, the verb cluster *continue to be* could be replaced by *are*.

Box 9.5 Use of verbs (underlined) in an introduction section

People who <u>are</u> overweight or obese <u>are</u> at increased risk of <u>developing</u> many illnesses including hypertension, cardiovascular disease and non-insulin dependent diabetes. However, many adults <u>continue to be</u> overweight. In 1995, results from the National Nutrition Survey in Australia <u>suggested</u> that 63% of men and 47% of women <u>were</u> either overweight or obese.

Despite the impact of excess body weight on health, self-perception of body mass in the general population <u>has not been</u> properly investigated. The only information <u>comes</u> from small, unrepresentative samples of women, particularly younger women, or from national studies in which self-reported weights <u>may be</u> unreliable. Until reliable information of self-perceptions of body mass <u>is</u> collected, it <u>is</u> difficult to design effective weight loss intervention strategies.

In 1998, we <u>conducted</u> a large cross-sectional survey of adults in which we accurately <u>measured</u> height and weight. In this paper, we <u>report</u> information about adults' perceptions of their own body mass.

Split infinitives

> *If you think a sentence will be more emphatic, clear or rhythmical, split your infinitive – there is no reason in logic or grammar for avoiding it. (Some sentences) seem better split than not. Take care though, lest the gap between "to" and the verb word becomes too great, as the reader could lose track of the meaning.*
>
> Martin Cutts[5]

It is common mantra that infinitive verbs need to be treated with great care and certainly should not be split. Most of us know this rule and yet may not know what an infinitive is.

Table 9.4 shows how to recognise infinitive and split infinitives. The most easily recognised infinitives are verbs that begin with *to* as in *to write*. There are also other types of infinitives that are recognisable as the last word in a verb cluster. For example, in the sentence *I must write* the word *must* is an auxiliary verb and *write* is the infinitive, which, because it does not appear with another word, is called a bare infinitive. In the examples that show split infinitives, the words *more than* splits into the centre of the infinitive *to double*. In the following example, the word *carefully* is placed between the auxiliary verb and its infinitive, so this is similarly split.

Reference books on English grammar restrict split infinitives to word(s) used between *to* and the verb because "infinitive" refers to the *to*—form.[6]

Unsplitting an infinitive often requires reorganising the sentence. In the first example of a split infinitive in Table 9.4, the sentence could be reorganised as *I want to make the review*

Table 9.4 Recognising infinitives and split infinitives.

Type	Example
"To" infinitives	I would like *to write* this paper
Bare infinitives	I *must write* this paper
Split infinitives	I want *to more than double* the length of the review that I am writing
	I want you *to carefully consider* my amendments to your paper
Infinitives that are not split	I happily *began to write* the journal article

that I am writing more than double its present length. Of course, not everyone agrees that infinitives should not be split and many great writers have knowingly and successfully split their infinitives. Indeed, we have split some infinitives in this book.

Who does what?

> *Verbs add drama to a random grouping of other words, producing an event, a happening, an exciting moment.*
>
> Constance Hale[7]

Many verbs can only be used if the subject is human. It is important that these verbs are not used to attribute an action to a non-human subject that cannot actually perform that action. Table 9.5 shows some of the verbs that can only have a human subject and some of the verbs that can have a human or non-human subject. In writing about your *study* or your *results* or any other non-human nouns associated with your research, you cannot use any of the verbs in the left-hand side of the table. However, the verbs in the right-hand side of the table are freely available for your use.

When you choose a verb, it is important not to suggest that your study can do the research all by itself. For example, in a sentence such as *A study that collects information from the time of diagnosis is needed,* the verb *collects* cannot be used with the noun *study.* The sentence is more correctly written as *A study is needed in which data can be collected from the time of diagnosis.* This satisfies the rules of verb use shown in

Table 9.5 Examples of verbs taking a human subject only or human/non-human subject.

Human subject only	Human or non-human subject
Observe	Show
Record	Demonstrate
Compare	Indicate
Identify	Suggest
Describe	Support
See	Confirm
Speculate	Imply
Conclude	Need
Believe	
Know	
Collect	
Aim	

Table 9.5 and puts the phrases in the order in which the reader needs to receive them. In this way, the study is treated as a tool that we use to test a hypothesis and is not ascribed the powers of a researcher.

Similar errors are apparent in phrases such as *This study seeks to ...*, *This study will determine ...*, *This research aims to ...* and even *This study has looked at ...*. The latter image is quite absurd. This erroneous assignment of power is not limited to the world of science. In a recent TV documentary, the commentator waxed lyrical with *As winter releases its icy grip ...*. Such licence may be acceptable for poetry and the media but must not be used in scientific writing, which should be limited to describing facts. Box 9.6 shows some examples of common verb misuses and their corrections.

Box 9.6 Can the noun do that?

1. ✖ To gather this information, a study <u>which collects information</u> from the time of diagnosis is needed
   ✓ To collect this information, <u>data must be collected</u> from the time of diagnosis

2. ✖ <u>This study aims to detect</u> a relation between disease severity and clinical outcome
   ✓ <u>The aim of conducting this study was to investigate</u> whether clinical outcome is related to disease severity

(continued)

---

3 ✖ Previous studies <u>have found that</u> most of the increase in the prevalence of asthma has occurred in children
   ✓ Most of the increase in the prevalence of asthma <u>has been</u> in children

4 ✖ Previous <u>studies have looked at</u> an association between family history of disease and clinical outcome
   ✓ Previous <u>researchers have investigated</u> the association between family history of disease and clinical outcome

5 ✖ <u>Houses that used evaporative coolers for air conditioning</u> had over three times more Der p I in both bed and floor dust
   ✓ <u>Houses with evaporative air coolers</u> had over three times more DerpI in both bed and floor dust

6 ✖ <u>This study aims to measure</u> the prevalence of several childhood illnesses
   ✓ <u>The aim of conducting this study is to measure</u> the prevalence of several childhood illnesses

7 ✖ <u>Table 2 compares</u> exposure levels in the cases and controls
   ✓ <u>Table 2 shows</u> exposure levels in the case and control groups

8 ✖ Final estimates of effect were made using a logistic regression model <u>that adjusted for</u> seasonality and overdispersion
   ✓ We used logistic regression to calculate the final estimates of effect <u>which were adjusted</u> for seasonality and overdispersion

Notes on verbs

Verbs should not be interchanged with prepositions. For example, in the sentence *Participants with allergy who have seasonal symptoms* is better written as *Participants who have allergy with seasonal symptoms* so that the verb is placed correctly in the sentence. Verbs and nouns also get muddled when their spelling is similar. For example, *affect* is usually a verb and *effect* is usually a noun. An example of the correct use of both is in the sentence *When you <u>affect</u> something, you have an <u>effect</u> on it.*

Students often ask whether it is correct to use *may* or *might* in scientific text to express whether something is possible, for example as in *Babies who are allergic <u>may</u> develop severe skin rash.* Sometimes, *might* is construed as describing a possibility that is more remote than *may.* However, as far as we can tell, there is no difference in meaning between *may* and *might* when they are used in the sense of possibility. Of course, *may* can sometimes indicate permission and the two words can be used interchangeably.

A verb that is often used in scientific writing is *performed*. For example, a researcher may write that *Lung function tests were performed in 21 infants*. The primary meaning of *performed* is in the context of acting. To be correct, it is more straightforward to write that *Twenty-one infants had lung function tests* or *Twenty-one infants underwent lung function testing*.

One final note on the use of verbs is that sentences ending with a verb tend to be ugly. For example, the sentences *We found that atopy to cat dander was not associated with asthma but that atopy to house dust mites was* and *Children who live in rural areas have a lower prevalence of allergy than those who do not* do not make pleasant reading. Sentences that have their verbs in the centre where they belong in a classical subject–verb–object sentence are much easier to read. Rewriting the first sentence as *Atopy to house dust mites, but not to cat dander, was associated with asthma* is much nicer. In the second sentence, the ending *than those who do not* can be deleted since this meaning is understood.

Adverbs

In "Yesterday, all my troubles were so far away" the adverb "yesterday" tells when Paul McCartney's troubles seemed so far away.

Constance Hale[7]

Adverbs are words that are used to modify verbs, adjectives, or other adverbs. A way to think about adverbs is in terms of the questions that they answer such as When? Where? What? Why? and How? Thus, adverbs can describe time (for example, *immediately, now, soon*), place (*here, there, everywhere*), manner (*boldly, hopefully, ideally*) or degree (*quickly, quite, very*). In these examples, many adverbs end with "-ly", although not all "-ly" words are adverbs. For example, some words such as *westerly* or *friendly* are adjectives.

Sentences can begin with an adverb that is followed by a comma and which sets the tone of the sentence. For example, in the sentence *Ideally, your references will have been entered into an electronic filing database* the word *ideally* is an adverb that modifies the verb *to enter*. The adverbs that cause most problems are those that merely repeat the meaning of the verb. Obvious examples that come to mind are *shouted <u>loudly,</u> ran <u>quickly</u>* and *mixed <u>together</u>*. In these phrases, the adverb is a tautology. The sentence *We are prospectively measuring growth and diet* is better written as *We are measuring growth and diet in a prospective study* with the adverb *prospectively* changed to its correct function as an adjective to describe the study design.

Conjunctions (joining words), such as *however, although,* and *thus,* are adverb hybrids. As explained in Chapter 8, these words are used to link sentences together. Other words can act as either an adverb or a conjunction. For example, in the sentence *He has only just arrived* the word *only* is an adverb because it modifies the verb *to arrive*. However, in the sentence *I would write the paper only I have several tasks to complete first,* the word *only* is used as a conjunction to join the descriptive clause *I have several tasks to complete first* to the main clause. In rewriting text, it sometimes helps to identify the function that each word has in a sentence.

Whilst it is often important to include modifiers in your sentences, they should not be used to rescue a sentence. In tight writing, adverbs are best avoided by choosing a verb that doesn't need modifying. It is preferable to choose nouns and verbs that are strong and that convey most of the message without the support of words that qualify them. In Box 9.7, the adverbs used in Box 3.2 from Chapter 3 are underlined. Only three adverbs are used in these paragraphs, all of which end in the telltale "-ly". The adverb *particularly* is an adverb hybrid that is being used as a conjunction. You could argue that the clause in which the adverb *accurately* is used would be better written as *in which we made accurate measurements of height and weight,* which correctly uses *accurate* as an adjective to describe the noun *measurements*.

Box 9.7 Use of adverbs (underlined) in an introduction section

People who are overweight or obese are at increased risk of developing many illnesses including hypertension, cardiovascular disease and non-insulin dependent diabetes. However, many adults continue to be overweight. In 1995, results from the National Nutrition Survey in Australia suggested that 63% of men and 47% of women were either overweight or obese.

Despite the impact of excess body weight on health, self-perception of body mass in the general population has not been <u>properly</u> investigated. The only information comes from small, unrepresentative samples of women, <u>particularly</u> younger women, or from national studies in which self-reported weights may be unreliable. Until reliable information of self-perceptions of body mass is collected, it is difficult to design effective weight loss intervention strategies.

In 1998, we conducted a large cross-sectional survey of adults in which we <u>accurately</u> measured height and weight. In this paper, we report information about adults' perceptions of their own body mass.

Pronouns and determiners

Keeping pronouns straight is as important to writing as keeping a firm hand on the rudder is to sailing. Your biggest problems with pronouns will come if you lose sight of the antecedent: when a pronoun drifts away from its antecedent, the entire message get lost at sea.

Constance Hale[8]

A pronoun is a word that is a proxy for a noun. In scientific writing, we need to be very direct so there is little use for proxies that mean something else. However, if you do use a pronoun, it must have a clear noun that it refers to. In this section, we discuss some tricks to identify and avoid the use of pronouns. Pronouns are best avoided where possible because they cause havoc when the noun they refer to is not clear. Table 9.6 lists the primary pronouns and shows the forms that are used as the subject or object in a sentence.

Pronouns that are used to indicate possession are called "determiners" or sometimes "demonstrative adjectives" because they act like an adjective in that they appear immediately before the noun that they modify. In the sentence, *After the woman had completed <u>her</u> tests, she collected <u>her</u> results*, the word *her* is used as a determiner. Table 9.7 shows the major sets of words that are pronouns or determiners in addition to the primary pronouns shown in Table 9.6.

Table 9.6 Pronouns that can be subject (the nominative case) or object (the objective case) in a sentence.

Subject or nominative case	Object or objective case
I	Me
You	You
He	Him
She	Her
It	It
We	Us
You	You
They	Them

Table 9.7 Major sets of pronouns and determiners.

Primary pronouns or determiners	my, mine myself, herself, himself, ourselves
Wh-pronouns or determiners	what, whose who, which whatever, whichever
Indefinite pronouns or determiners	some, somebody, anybody, any, anyone, anything, everyone, none, nothing few, many, all
Demonstrative pronouns	this, that these, those, they

The indefinite pronouns are words that refer to unspecified persons or unspecified objects. The demonstrative pronouns can be singular, i.e. *this* or *that*, or can be plural, i.e. *these* or *those*. In general, *this* and *these* indicate closeness and *that* and *those* indicate remoteness.

In the jargon of grammar, the noun to which a pronoun refers is called the "antecedent" because it comes before the pronoun in the text. A pronoun and its antecedent must always agree in person, number and gender. For example, in the sentence *After the woman had completed her tests, <u>she</u> collected her results*, the pronoun *she* refers to the antecedent *woman* and is therefore singular and female. The two pronouns *her*, which are also singular and female, are examples of pronouns used to indicate possession and are therefore determiners.

Whenever you use a pronoun, always double check that its meaning is not ambiguous. Most importantly, the clarity of a sentence should not be compromised by a pronoun losing sight of its antecedent. Some examples of pronouns that have been "let on the loose"[8] are shown in Box 9.8. In the first example, the pronoun *they* actually refers to *febrile seizures* but has been placed too far away from this antecedent so that it mistakenly appears to be referring to the noun *illnesses*. A similar problem occurs in example 2, where the reader has to backtrack a long way to find the antecedent.

In the third example, the overload of the use of the pronoun *those* leaves the reader bewildered about what each of them is referring to. If you are ever tempted to use the word *those*, it is usually a clear sign that the sentence should be rewritten quickly. In the final example, *those* appears to refer to *wild type mites* which doesn't make sense because wild type mites cannot come from culture.

Box 9.8 Pronouns on the loose[8]

1 ✘ Febrile seizures are the commonest form of neurological illnesses. <u>They</u> occur between the ages of six months to five years and present with seizures, usually the convulsive type, in association with fever

   ✓ Febrile seizures are the commonest form of seizure disorder in children aged from six months to five years. Such seizures are usually convulsive and are usually associated with fever

2 ✘ Comparisons of the prevalence of asthma have been restricted to <u>those</u> where identical methods were used

   ✓ In comparing the prevalence of asthma, we have only selected studies in which identical methods were used

3 ✘ There was no difference in a family history of diabetes between <u>those</u> with complete follow up data and <u>those</u> without. <u>Those</u> with complete follow up data tended to have mothers with more years of education than <u>those</u> without

   ✓ There was a similar prevalence of a family history of diabetes in the participants and in the children who were lost to follow up, but the mothers of participants tended to have more years of education

4 ✘ Wild type mites and <u>those</u> from culture can differ in their responses to temperature and humidity

   ✓ Wild type and cultured mites can differ in their responses to temperature and humidity

There is absolutely no need to use a pronoun determiner when a shorter, definite article is better. For example, in the sentence *Only those children whose parents gave written consent were included in the study*, the determiner *those* is much better replaced by the definite article *the* and the sentence written as *Only the children with parental consent were studied*.

Two golden rules of scientific writing are: never use the word *those* and severely limit use of *these* and *they*. The use of the word *those* is highly indicative of a lazy sentence structure and is usually a clear signal of a sentence that is foggy at best, and grammatically incorrect at worst.

Another pronoun that should be avoided if possible is the word *it*. The best rule about using the word *it* is to never use this word to begin a sentence. *It*, which is sometimes referred to in a derogatory sense as the "ubiquitous it", has few uses in unambiguous writing. Beginning a sentence with this pronoun usually leaves readers scanning the previous sentence to find what the mystery *It* refers to. In the text *Lack of exercise is a specific indictor of high blood pressure. It is associated with breathlessness on exertion and long term heart disease*, the *it* that begins the second sentence appears to refer to the antecedent noun cluster *high blood pressure* but in fact is referring to *lack of exercise*. This type of problem is easily solved with a quick rewrite.

Of course there is always the exception to the rule and some *it* words that begin sentences do not need an antecedent. For example, in a sentence such as *It is important that you use the correct statistical test*, the pronoun *it* is called an "anticipatory" it. This pronoun is used to balance a sentence when the most important part, i.e. *that you use the correct statistical test*, is used as a clause at the end of a sentence rather than as a noun cluster at the beginning. The sentence could be written as *Using the correct statistical test is important*. Both sentences are fine; your choice just depends on the context in which you are writing.

From the example shown in Box 3.2 in Chapter 3, only four words remain that are not nouns, verbs, adverbs or prepositions: the two words *that* in paragraph 1 and *it* in paragraph 2 are correctly used pronouns. In the third paragraph, the words *this* and *their* are pronouns used as determiners.

Notes on pronouns

The use of a singular noun with a plural pronoun is a terrible grammatical style that is creeping into scientific writing in order to avoid the use of gender specific pronouns such as his and hers. Box 9.9 shows some examples of sentences in which a plural pronoun is incorrectly used. The simplest way to solve this problem is to make the noun plural, as shown in examples 1 and 3, or to make the pronoun singular as shown in example 2. Other methods are to leave out the pronoun altogether, repeat the noun, or recast the sentence using an alternative pronoun or no pronoun at all. If at all possible, never use the term *his/her* to avoid a gender specific meaning.

Box 9.9 Avoiding gender-specific pronouns

1 ✗ Mentoring is a process in which a senior researcher shares their experience with a junior researcher
  ✓ Mentoring is a process in which senior researchers share their experiences with junior researchers

2 ✗ A team leader may select a junior researcher because they have shown insight into some of the research processes
  ✓ A team leader may select a junior researcher who has shown insight into some of the research processes

3 ✗ Publishing research results has benefits to the team leader and his/her research unit
  ✓ Publishing research results has benefits to team leaders and their departments

---

Conjunctions and prepositions

Words that help point us in the right direction (prepositions such as on, about and around) sometimes give confusing signals. The reader might take an unnecessary detour or even a wrong turn. Notice how the preposition on *can give a sentence two very different meanings: Jon wrote a book on Mount Everest.*

Patricia O'Conner[2]

Conjunctions are the words that are used to link phrases, clauses, or sentences to one another. Conjunctions act like the glue that holds your writing together. Words such as *and, but, or, yet, so, either/or* are commonly used conjunctions.

On the other hand, prepositions are words that point us in a direction. Prepositions are easy to spot because they are the small words such as *as, in, on, of,* and *among*. These small words can cause big problems, so ensure that the direction in which your preposition points your reader is correct. For example, participants are recruited *into* a study not *onto* a study, and you conduct a *study of diabetes* not a *study in diabetes*. Also, people *take* medications rather than being *on* them. The sentence *In children who survived to 5 years, 11·2% had a disability* is better than *Among children who survived to 5 years, 11·2% had a disability*. Not only is the first sentence shorter, it is more correct because you mean the prevalence in all of the children not just some of them.

When you use a preposition, visualise the direction it is signalling and ask yourself if it is appropriate. Cats sit *on* mats, go *into* rooms, are part *of* a family, or roam *amongst* the flowers. The meanings of some commonly used prepositions are shown in Table 9.8. If you are unsure about the use of a preposition, ask yourself what the cat would do.

Sometimes sentences have prepositions slotted in for no apparent reason. For example, in the title *A prospective study of walking as compared with aerobic exercise in the treatment of obesity*, the preposition *as* fulfils no function except that of cluttering up an otherwise clear title. In the title *Infant and maternal outcomes in the pregnancies of women with asthma*, the preposition *in* is not quite right because an outcome cannot be in anything, although it can be used in a study. The title would be better written as *Infant and maternal outcomes in a study of pregnant women with asthma* or as *Infant and pregnancy outcomes of mothers with asthma*. The second version is both shorter and has only one necessary preposition.

In the sentence *The value of your property as at 8ᵗʰ August was $700 000*, the prepositions "as at" are best replaced by the single preposition *on*. In phrases that begin with *All of the*, the word *of* can be omitted. Sentences do not need to be written with preposition overload.

Box 9.10 shows some examples of how sentences become clearer and more straightforward when the prepositions are

Table 9.8 Prepositions and their common meanings.

Preposition	Meaning
in, into	Inclusion or position within defined limits, as in *We enrolled participants in our study*
on	Supported by or covering, as in *The equipment was on the bench*
among, amongst	In the middle of or between, as in *There is honour among thieves.* Remember to use *between* for two things and *among* for more than two things, unless referring to exact position or precise individual relationships for example, *consensus guidelines between France, Germany, and Italy*
with	Together with, as in *This goes with that*
as	Used to express degree or manner, as in *It is not as easy as you think*
of	Indicates a relation as in *Many of the participants withdrew from the study*

removed. In example 1, the preposition *with* is used incorrectly to mean *as a result of.* The intention of the sentence is not to say that, the pain occurs concurrently with poor posture or incorrect lifting but rather that pain occurs following poor posture or incorrect lifting. In example 2, *as to* is clumsy and *of* is better. This sentence is a good example of not giving information in the correct order so that we have to read all the way to the end of the sentence to find out that we should find the question interesting.

The double use of *with* and *to* in example 3 and of *as* in sentence 4 are clear indicators that better writing is needed. In example 5, the phrase *due to* is used to mean *because.* Whenever you see the word *due* as used in example 5, remind yourself that it is best limited to describing trains and buses.

Box 9.10 Being careful with prepositions

1 ✘ Back pain can occur with poor sitting or standing posture or with incorrect lifting techniques

  ✓ Back pain can result from poor posture or incorrect lifting techniques

(continued)

2 ✖ The question <u>as to</u> whether RSV infection induces a Th1 or Th2 inflammatory response is interesting
  ✓ The question <u>of</u> whether RSV infection induces a Th1 or Th2 inflammatory response is interesting
  ✓ It would be interesting to know whether RSV infection induces a Th1 or Th2 response

3 ✖ The risk of being diagnosed <u>with</u> asthma in children <u>with</u> negative skin prick tests is strongly related <u>to</u> exposure <u>to</u> early childhood infections
  ✓ The risk of non-allergic children being diagnosed with asthma is strongly related to exposure to early childhood infections
  ✓ Non-allergic children are more likely to have asthma if they have a respiratory infection during early childhood

4 ✖ The aim is <u>to</u> determine whether paediatric and adolescent patients <u>with</u> Crohn's disease have <u>as</u> severe protein malnutrition <u>as</u> patients with anorexia nervosa
  ✓ The aim of conducting this study is to assess whether protein malnutrition is of similar severity in patients with Crohn's disease or with anorexia nervosa

5 ✖ The remaining children were not available <u>due to</u> residence outside the study area
  ✓ The remaining children where not studied <u>because</u> they lived outside the study area

Box 9.11 shows the conjunctions and prepositions used in Box 3.2. Although up to four prepositions are used in some sentences, they are all necessary to indicate direction.

Box 9.11 Use of prepositions (underlined) and conjunctions (bold type) in an introduction section

People who are overweight **or** obese are <u>at</u> increased risk <u>of</u> developing many illnesses **including** hypertension, cardiovascular disease **and** non-insulin dependent diabetes. **However**, many adults continue to be overweight. <u>In</u> 1995, results <u>from</u> the National Nutrition Survey <u>in</u> Australia suggested that 63% of men **and** 47% <u>of</u> women were **either** overweight **or** obese.

Despite the impact <u>of</u> excess body weight <u>on</u> health, self-perception <u>of</u> body mass <u>in</u> the general population has not been properly investigated. The only information comes <u>from</u> small, unrepresentative samples <u>of</u> women, particularly younger women, **or** <u>from</u> national studies <u>in</u> which self-reported weights may be unreliable. **Until** reliable information <u>of</u> self-perceptions <u>of</u> body mass is collected, it is difficult to design effective weight loss intervention strategies.

<u>In</u> 1998, we conducted a large cross-sectional survey of adults <u>in</u> which we accurately measured height **and** weight. <u>In</u> this paper, we report information <u>about</u> adults' perceptions <u>of</u> their own body mass.

Phrases

People do not think in single words as a rule … . Mostly we think in groups of words, and we certainly need to write in groups of words.

Elizabeth Murphy[9]

Groups of words fall into phrases or clauses, usually depending on whether or not a verb is present. A phrase is a small group of words that cannot stand alone and that does not meet the requirements of being a complete sentence. Because phrases are used to explain little parts of the sentence in more detail, they have been described as *simple word groupings – bits of organised thought that are part of the complete idea behind a sentence.*[10]

The following two sentences contain the phrases *under my chair, through the gate*, and *down the road: I left my book <u>under my chair;</u> I walked <u>through the gate</u> and <u>down the road</u>.*

Phrases can be prepositional, verb, or noun phrases as shown in Table 9.9. There is not much to say about phrases except that they should always be short and snappy.

Table 9.9 Types of phrases.

Type of phrase	Example
Prepositional phrase	on the chair behind the door in the book
Verb phrase	has been seen to be done was reported
Noun phrase	the long and winding road longitudinal cohort studies important confounders

Clauses

No subject though is so complicated that it can't be explained in clear English. If you can't explain something to another person, maybe – just maybe – you don't quite understand it yourself.

Patricia O'Conner[2]

Because clauses have a subject, a verb, and an object, they have more impact in a sentence than a phrase. Clauses can form a whole sentence. Alternatively, two or more clauses can be joined together by a conjunction or separated by punctuation marks to make a sentence. Clauses that are known as independent clauses can stand alone but other clauses known as dependent clauses need an independent clause for support.

When two independent clauses are joined together, the resulting sentence is called a "compound" sentence. For example, the sentence *We used electronic scales to measure weight and we used a stadiometer to measure height* is a compound sentence because the word *and* could be replaced by a full stop and both short sentences could stand alone. The most common conjunctions that are used to join two clauses are *and*, *but,* and *or*. The conjunctions that are commonly used to join a dependent clause to an independent clause are *because, as, if, who, which, when,* and *where*.

Table 9.10 shows examples of types of clauses and their nomenclature. In the example of an independent clause, *I would like to write a book* forms the entire sentence, whereas the second example has two independent clauses joined with the conjunction *but*.

Dependent clauses are often adjectival clauses. In the same way that adjectives are "describing words", adjectival clauses are "describing clusters of words". In the examples of dependent clauses in Table 9.10, the first sentence has an independent clause and a dependent clause introduced by the conjunction *when*. In the next sentence, the dependent clause, *that I would like to write*, begins with a pronoun and is embedded within an independent clause. The last example shows a prepositional clause that is clearly indicated by beginning with the preposition *into*.

Table 9.10 Examples of types of clauses.

Alternative nomenclatures	Characteristics	Examples
Independent, main, or restrictive clause	Can stand alone as a complete sentence	<u>I would like to write a book</u>
	Is not parenthetic and does not need commas	<u>I would like to write a book</u> but <u>I do not want to write a journal article</u>
	Can be joined together with one of the conjunctions: *and, but, or*	
Dependent, subordinate, non-restrictive, adjectival, or commenting clause	Cannot stand alone as a complete sentence	I would like to write a book <u>when I can find time to do it</u>
	Sometimes needs a comma to cordon it off from the independent clause	The book, <u>which I will be working on soon,</u> will be published next year
	Adds information to a sentence	The book <u>that I would like to write</u> is being considered for publication
	Usually introduced with a conjunction such as *because, who, when, which, where, if, as, although*	<u>Although I would like to write a book</u>, I cannot find time to do it
Prepositional clause	Consists of a preposition followed by its object	We recruited 50 participants <u>into our research study</u>

Table 9.11 shows how simple messages can be rewritten using a variety of different types of phrases and clauses. All of the sentences have an independent clause by necessity. In all except the first sentence, other phrases and dependent clauses modify the independent clause.

The independent clauses that were used in Box 3.2 in Chapter 3 are underlined in Box 9.12. The main messages of the text are carried in these clauses. The remainder of the text is comprised of dependent clauses, adjectival phrases,

Table 9.11 Examples of phrases and clauses.

Sentence	Components
The fox jumped over the dog	Independent clause using a prepositional phrase *over the dog*
The quick, brown fox jumped over the lazy dog	Independent clause using a noun phrase *the quick brown fox*, a verb *jumped* and a prepositional phrase *over the lazy dog*
The fox that jumped over the lazy dog was quick and was brown	Independent clause *the fox was quick and was brown* embedded with a dependent essential adjectival clause *that jumped over the lazy dog*
The fox, which was quick and was brown, jumped over the lazy dog	Independent clause embedded with a dependent non-essential adjectival clause
The lazy dog was jumped over by a quick, brown fox	Independent clause with only one verb
The lazy dog was jumped over by a fox,which was quick and was brown	Independent clause followed by a dependent non-essential adjectival clause
The lazy dog was jumped over by the fox that killed the chicken	Independent clause followed by a dependent essential adjectival clause

and conjunctions, which are there simply to add detail and create flow.

Box 9.12 Use of independent clauses (underlined) in an introduction section

Introduction

People who are overweight or obese are at increased risk of developing many illnesses including hypertension, cardiovascular disease and non-insulin dependent diabetes. However, many adults continue to be overweight. In 1995, results from the National Nutrition Survey in Australia suggested that 63% of men and 47% of women were either overweight or obese.

Despite the impact of excess body weight on health, self-perception of body mass in the general population has not been properly investigated. The only information comes from small, unrepresentative

> samples of women, particularly younger women, <u>or from national studies in which self-reported weights may be unreliable</u>. Until reliable information of self-perceptions of body mass is collected, <u>it is difficult to design effective weight loss intervention strategies</u>.
>
> In 1998, <u>we conducted a large cross-sectional survey of adults</u> in which we accurately measured height and weight. In this paper, <u>we report information about adults' perceptions of their own body mass</u>.

Which and that

> *The use of "which" for "that" is common in written and spoken language. ("Let us now go even unto Bethlehem and see this thing which is come to pass.") Occasionally "which" seems preferable to "that" as in the sentence from the Bible … . But it would be a convenience to all if these two pronouns were used with precision. Careful writers, watchful for small inconveniences, go "which"-hunting, remove the defining "whiches", and by doing so, improve their work.*
>
> William Strunk Jr[3]

The words *which* and *that* are pronouns that are commonly used to begin adjectival clauses, but deciding when to use each one sometimes causes problems. The rules to decide when to use *that* or *which* are grounded in the formal construction of sentences. *That* is used to begin an *essential adjectival clause*. Essential clauses are fundamental to the meaning of the sentence, immediately follow the word that they modify, and do not need any punctuation to separate them from the remainder of the sentence. In the sentence, *I would like to show you the book <u>that</u> I am writing,* the clause *that I am writing* is essential and adjectival, and therefore begins with *that*. Of course you can let your electronic grammar checker decide whether to use *which* or *that* for you, but it is much better to have a clear idea about which is the correct word to use rather than let your computer make executive decisions for you.

The word *which* is used to begin a "non-essential adjectival clause". Non-essential clauses also immediately follow the word that they modify but merely add interest to the sentence. For this reason, non-essential clauses are usually enclosed by punctuation marks because they can be omitted from the sentence without influencing the main message. In the sentence *I would like to show you my book, <u>which</u> is now on sale in the bookshops*, the clause *which is now on sale in the bookshops* is dependent, non-essential, and adjectival.

In recognising when to use *which* and when to use *that* you can structure your sentences accordingly in the knowledge that if the grammar checker doesn't question your choice of words, you will. In Box 3.2 there are only two uses of the word *which*, and both are used in conjunction with *in* to begin adjectival clauses. There is only one use of the word *that*. There are no examples of *which* or *that* used in the classical sense without a preposition to begin a clause.

After the nouns, adjectives, verbs, adverbs, pronouns, prepositions and conjunctions in Box 3.2 are identified, all that remain are the numbers, that is *1995*, *63%* and *47%* in the first paragraph, and *1998* in the final paragraph.

Grammar matters

Please write in a clear, direct and active style.

BMJ house style (www.bmj.com)

The few simple rules of grammar that you need to know are summarised in Box 9.13. With these rules under your belt, you should be able to classify types of words into their nomenclature, write correctly, and understand why reviewers suggest that you rewrite your sentences. The good news is that once you are comfortable with these rules, writing will become a much simpler task. All you will need to do is analyse the sentences that are giving you trouble, separate them into their basic components, and decide how you want to remedy the problems. With these skills, you will also become a valuable reviewer.

Box 9.13 Grammar choices

Check that you are not using any nouns as adjectives
Ensure that verb tenses match noun plurals
Watch out for sneaky plurals
Ensure that your verbs can take a non-human subject
Choose short verb forms and use the active voice

Avoid pronouns on the loose
Never use 'those' and be careful with *these* and *they*
Participants are people who deserve the correct pronoun
Minimise the number of prepositions
Do you mean *as, in, on, among,* or *due*?

Acknowledgements

The Shaw quote has been produced with permission from Horvitz, LA ed. *The Quotable Scientist*. New York: McGraw-Hill Companies, 2000 (p 18). The O'Conner quotes: excerpts from *Words Fail Me: What Everyone Who Writes Should Know About Writing*, copyright © 1999 by Patricia O'Conner have been reprinted by permission of Harcourt, Inc. All other referenced quotes have been produced with permission.

References

1 Lamott A. *Some instructions on writing and life*. London: Anchor Books, 1994; p 151.
2 O'Conner P. *Words fail me*. London: Harcourt, 1999; pp 9, 59, 65, 118.
3 Strunk Jr W. *The elements of style*. New York: Allyn and Bacon, 2000; pp xvii, 59.
4 Hale C. Verbs. In: *Sin and syntax*. New York: Broadway Books, 1999; p 55.
5 Cutts M. *The plain English guide*. Oxford: Oxford University Press, 1996; pp 96, 97.
6 Greenbaum S. *Oxford English grammer*. Oxford: Oxford University Press, 1996.
7 Hale C. *Sin and syntax*. New York: Broadway Books, 1999; pp 44, 88.
8 Hale C. Pronouns. In: *Sin and syntax*. New York: Broadway Books, 1999; pp 42–54.
9 Murphy E. *Effective writing*. London: Longman Cheshire Pty Ltd, 1989.
10 Hale C. Phrases and clauses. In: *Sin and syntax*. New York: Broadway Books, 1999; pp 169–81.

10: Word choice

Like all art forms, writing is a craft and takes practice.
The sooner you start, the sooner you will become more
proficient in choosing your words and arranging them on
the page in a way that best expresses what you have to
say. It's not easy, but the effort is immensely rewarding.

Irina Dunn[1]

> The objectives of this chapter are to understand how to:
> - choose the correct words
> - avoid the wrong words
> - write neat sentences that mean what you want them to mean

Because most of us think in groups of words, we need to be
able to write in groups of words for the benefit of our readers.
To achieve this, every scientist needs to become something of
a wordsmith. The words that we choose for our purpose must
be selected and assembled using correct syntax and grammar.
In this chapter, we explain how to choose words that are
appropriate for scientific writing and how to avoid some
common mistakes.

Label consistently

The reader's job is to follow the author's thinking and to
agree or disagree; it is not to decode and reconstruct the
paper. Thus, if you want your readers to get your message,
you will have to make it abundantly clear to them.

Mimi Zeiger[2]

When you are writing about the participants whom you
enrolled in your study, the equipment that you used, the
outcomes you measured, or the results that you found,
always use terms in your paper consistently. This seems a fairly

obvious thing to say, but it is surprising how often writers freely switch between different terms to mean the same thing. For example, it is common to see the words *children, participants, respondents, persons, cases,* and *controls* all used interchangeably. However, chopping and changing suggests that you are talking about many different groups of participants and leads to confusion. The example in Box 10.1 shows how much clearer the text becomes when standardised terms are used to describe the study participants. In the corrected version, the term *children* to describe the study group is defined and used consistently.

Box 10.1 Standardising terms

✗ Meningococcal disease is most prevalent in <u>children under 2 years of age</u>. Approximately 400 healthy <u>toddlers</u> aged 12–15 months will be enrolled in this trial. <u>Children</u> will be randomised to receive either the new vaccine or a standard immunisation schedule. <u>Children</u> who are randomised to the control group will be offered the new vaccine at completion of the study.

✓ Meningococcal disease is most prevalent in <u>children under 2 years of age</u>. Approximately 400 healthy <u>children</u> aged 12–15 months will be enrolled in this trial. <u>Children</u> will be randomised to receive either the new vaccine or a standard immunisation schedule. <u>Children</u> who are randomised to the control group will be offered the new vaccine at completion of the study.

If you use different terms, they should mean different things and should be afforded separate definitions accordingly. Never be tempted to switch and change between different terms to describe the same outcome. For example, terms such as *atopy, allergic sensitisation, skin prick test positivity, allergen reactivity,* and *clinical allergy* all mean much the same thing but should not be used interchangeably. For indexing in databases such as MEDLINE®, it is better to select the most commonly used term, define it in the methods, and use it consistently. This is essential, even when quoting work from the literature in which the authors have used different terms to the ones you are using. For example, if you use the phrase *airway hyperresponsiveness*, then use it throughout and do not switch to *bronchial hyperreactivity* even if the researchers that you are quoting have used that term in their publications.

In standardising your terms, you need to select the appropriate term for your audience. If you are writing for a journal that specialises in allergic diseases, you would use the term *allergic rhinitis*, but if you were submitting the same paper to a general journal, you would use the term *hay fever*.

Even more importantly, you must always stick to the same point of view and use the same way of presenting data. It becomes quite confusing if you compare, for example, mortality rates in one group with survival rates in another. Also, do not compare risk factors for being underweight from one study with risk factors for being overweight from another study. This switching does not add interest but merely creates confusion. Always reword the work you are citing from other researchers' papers or rework their results if necessary, for example by changing mortality rates to survival rates, so that direct comparisons can be made.

Participants are people

> *Individual. A yucky word. Usually unnecessary. Use person or someone. Use individual only when you mean to distinguish an individual from a group or corporation.*
>
> Jack Lynch (www[1])

Participants are people not "things" and must always be described as such. The terms *subjects* and *individuals* are widely used, but the term *participants* is more politically correct because it reflects the role of people in the research process.[3] In clinical studies, it is important to refer to your participants as a *child* or a *patient* rather than a *case*. Be careful not to write sentences such as *Three cases were admitted to hospital*. A *case* is an episode of a disease; a *patient* is admitted to hospital.

It is also important to avoid pejorative terms such as *psychotics* or *schizophrenics* or other labelling of participants with their illness conditions, for example *asthmatics* or *diabetics*. For example, it is better to write *patients with diabetes* rather than *diabetic patients*. Also be careful not to dehumanise your participants by using the wrong noun or pronoun. For example, it is correct to write *participants <u>who</u>* and dehumanising to write *participants <u>that</u>* … .

Box 10.2 Using the correct pronouns or descriptors for participants

1. **✗** There was an increase in the proportion of children <u>that</u> reported having asthma over the study period
   ✓ There was an increase in the proportion of children who reported having asthma over the study period
   ✓ The proportion of children with asthma increased during the study period

2. **✗** At present we have two patients who are waiting for testing <u>that</u> would be suitable
   ✓ We have two patients waiting for testing who would be suitable

3. **✗** Neonatal infections affected babies <u>that</u> were smaller and born more premature
   ✓ Neonatal infections affected babies who were smaller and more premature
   ✓ Small and premature babies were more susceptible to neonatal infections

4. **✗** The wheezy infant remains <u>a conundrum</u> for both primary care teams and hospital paediatricians
   ✓ Treatment for wheezy infants remains a problem for primary care teams and hospital paediatricians
   ✓ Consensus treatment strategies for wheezy infants have not been developed

---

Box 10.2 shows how the wrong pronoun can sneak into a sentence and how it can be corrected. In example 1, the pronoun *that* refers to children and should be *who*. The sentence can also be shortened by replacing the phrase *who reported having* with the preposition *with*. In the second example, the pronoun *that* has become separated from its antecedent *patients*. When rejoined, it becomes clear that the pronoun is incorrect. In the third example the pronoun *who* is more appropriate than the word *that* and the sentence benefits from some rearrangement. In the fourth example, better words can be chosen to describe infants who present to hospital with a wheezing illness. It is the choice of appropriate treatment that is a challenge for physicians, not the infant itself.

Word choice

Never use a long word where a short one will do.

George Orwell (1903–1950)

In striving to write in an unambiguous way, you need to select the correct words. Ideally, use short words instead of long words. Sometimes long words are chosen in a thinly veiled attempt to appear academic. This is a big mistake. In fact, it is scholarly to choose a short word with the correct meaning rather than choose a long word with the wrong meaning. Most readers are busy people who will not appreciate having to find a dictionary to look up the meanings of obscure words or expressions. Making your readers work to decipher your message is an unfriendly act. Always choose short, clearly understood words. Table 10.1 shows some long words and word phrases with some alternative shorter versions that can be used.

Long words can clutter up a sentence. When you are choosing words, shorter ones are always better. For example, in the sentence *The centre has established an agreement with the museum to utilise either information collection system*, the phrase *has established an agreement* can be replaced with *has agreed*, and the term *utilise* with *use*. Thus, the sentence becomes simpler and more factually correct written as *The museum research committee has agreed that we can use their information collection systems*.

Sometimes a long word is not only long but may have the wrong meaning. For example *methodology* means *the study of methods* not *the methods used in the study*. If you use the word *dosage*, you mean the total amount of medication to be taken in a given period and not the amount to be taken at one time. Also, be clear about the different meanings of terms such as *prevalence* and *incidence* and do not use them interchangeably to mean the same thing.

Table 10.1 Using the correct word.

Long or incorrect version	Shorter or more correct version
Determine, detect	Assess, measure, investigate
Correlated (as an adjective or verb)	Associated
Due to the fact that, for the reason that, on account of, owing to the fact that, on the basis that	Because
Level (in solution)	Concentration
Documentation	Documents
Taken into consideration	Considered
Dosage	Dose
Elucidate, clarify	Explain
Functionality	Function
In the event of, in the eventuality of	If, when
Alleviate, moderate	Lessen, ease
Methodology	Methods
In close proximity to	Near
At the present moment, at this point in time	Now
The majority of	Most
Dyads	Pairs
Prioritise	Rank
Revealed	Show, found
Abuse (substance drug)	Misuse
Symptomatology, complaints, events, clinical picture	Symptoms
Terminology	Term
In order to	To
Usage, utilise	Use

Avoid emotive terms

> *Why is it that night falls but day breaks, and that the third hand on a watch is called the second hand?*

Taken from an internet bulletin board

Emotive terms are strictly off limits to scientific writers, who must be circumspect in their writing. We need to be factual and describe what we think or what we saw in a non-emotive way. In this quest, there is no place for jazzing up the human interest in your story. It is important to write about participants who *have back pain*, not participants who *suffer back pain*, or patients *who have HIV* or *who have anorexia nervosa* rather than patients who are *HIV sufferers* or *anorexia nervosa sufferers*. When the *P* value gets below 0·001, it is also best to limit your enthusiasm and describe something as a *strong* rather than a *powerful* risk factor. Some uses of emotive terms and suggestions of how to remedy them are shown in Box 10.3.

Box 10.3 Removing emotive terms

1 ✖ In order to <u>capture</u> clinically significant effect sizes with a power of 80% and a significance of 5%, 21 participants will be necessary in each group
  ✓ To show that the effects are significant at the 5% level with a power of 80%, 21 participants are required in each group

2 ✖ <u>Surprisingly,</u> it appears that feather pillows may protect against asthma
  ✓ There is good evidence that feather pillows protect against asthma

3 ✖ To plan effective interventions <u>to arrest</u> and reverse this trend, we need a better understanding of the risk factors that are involved
  ✓ To plan interventions to reverse this trend, we need a better understanding of the risk factors involved

4 ✖ <u>Unfortunately,</u> with our questionnaire, we had no way of knowing if subjects had wheeze only on exertion
  ✓ Our questionnaire did not allow us to identify participants who only experienced wheeze on exertion

5 ✖ It is unethical to mislead others by <u>broadcasting</u> results that turn out to be a mistake at a later date
  ✓ It is unethical to mislead others by reporting results that may turn out to be incorrect

6 ✖ Yet it is precisely those children <u>who reap the greatest benefit</u> from treatment and have the highest risk of treatment failure
  ✓ The children who may receive the greatest benefit from the treatment have a higher risk of treatment failure

---

A common word used is *reveal* as in *The present study <u>reveals</u> that more than half of the children studied were exposed to tobacco smoke in their homes*. *Reveal* is a funny word that suggests something was found perhaps by magic – like the rabbit in the hat when the magician sweeps his cloak away. Clothing is also described as *revealing* when it shows something that is probably best not shown. As such, the word *reveal* has connotations of disclosure rather than of demonstrating a scientific finding. It is much better to select a more straightforward word such as *showed* or *indicated* to describe your research results.

Because

> *In fact, really bad writing is rarely a matter of broken rules – editors can clean these up with a few pencil marks. It's more often the result of muddled thought. Bad writers consider long words more impressive than short ones, and the use of words like* usage *instead of* use *or* methodologies *instead of* methods *without knowing what they mean. The facts get buried under loads of useless words …*
>
> Jack Lynch(www[1])

In addition to avoiding long or emotive words, it is important to use small words correctly. In recent times, there has been an increasing trend to use the word *as* incorrectly. Examples of incorrect uses of the word *as* are shown in Box 10.4. In these sentences, the word *as* should be replaced by the word *because*. The *Oxford English Dictionary* describes the meaning of *because* as *for the reason that*. In the first example, the use of *cases* and *controls* to describe participants is dehumanising and also needs to be changed.

Box 10.4 Using "because" to mean "because"

✘ There may be bias <u>as</u> the cases were visited more regularly than the controls

✓ There may be bias because participants in the case group were visited more regularly than participants in the control group

✘ It is the general belief that the complex needs of these children, both in acute crisis and long term, are not being met <u>as</u> there is a lack of available and appropriate services

✓ The complex needs of these children, both in acute crisis and long term, are not being met because appropriate services are not available

---

The use of *as* to mean *because* began quite recently. This use is not listed in many dictionaries and is an exceedingly minor interpretation in others. The *Pocket Oxford English Dictionary* has only a very minor, subsidiary reference for *as* as follows:

> As. *"since, seeing that" as in "as he refuses, we can do nothing"*

This restores conviction. *Since* conveys an element of time, which is not quite correct for the scientific sentences in Box 10.4 and *seeing that* conveys an element of vision, which is not appropriate either. In the full *Oxford English Dictionary*, there is almost a half a page of microscopic text, as you might expect, to describe the correct meaning of *as* as an adverb in, for example, *They stood as one man*. However, half way down the second column, there is the following brief statement:

> As. *Of reason. It being the case that; inasmuch as; since*

This interpretation is reminiscent of the romantic writing of Jane Austen and does not validate the use of *as* to mean *because* in concise, scientific writing.

Scientific writing is the art of presenting research ideas clearly, documenting results precisely, and drawing implications correctly. In this, the word *because* is the superior word to use to convey reason, simply because its meaning is both clear and grammatically correct. The word *as* should only be used as an adverb, a relative adverb, or a relative pronoun in the following phrases in which *as* cannot be replaced by *because*:

- *it occurred as a result of*
- *as quiet as a mouse*
- *act as you think best*
- *he fulfilled his duty as a research assistant.*

Admittedly, constructs such as *as if* or *as cheap as* are new, stand-alone, colloquial statements. The words are used correctly in a grammatical sense, the minimalism conveys impact, and the unspoken ending is understood. In addition, our computers now ask *save as*, although they omit the question mark. It is interesting to ponder whether Shakespeare was correct when he wrote *As you like it*, but then artistic licence and scientific writing are entirely different.

Levels and concentrations

Using "level" to mean "concentration" may be colloquial but is hardly scientific. This is a matter that is best contemplated at leisure in the bath where you have time to consider the difference between the level of the water in the tub and the concentration of the bath salts in the water.

Jeff Aronson[4]

Another word that is widely misused in the scientific literature is the word *level* instead of *concentration*. For example, immunologists often describe *blood levels of protein* and *plasma levels of IgE* and allergists often describe *housedust mite allergen* levels, thus using the word *level* to mean *concentration*. *The Oxford English Dictionary* sheds some light on this problem. The meaning of the word *concentration* was a relatively late entry into the dictionary. Although the word *level* has been there a long time, none of its meanings has the sense of *concentration*.[4] If the word *concentration* is correct, then this word should be used. It is prudent to remember this the next time that you describe a concentration that you have measured in your study. It is better to be grammatically correct than follow new fashions in writing.

Untying the negatives

If the basic idea is too complicated to fit on a T-shirt, it's probably wrong.

Leon Lederman (physicist, 1984)

It is important to use negatives carefully and to use them only when they can't be avoided. Everyone knows the basic rule of mathematics that two negatives make a positive. The same rule applies to sentences. However, instead of using two negatives, it is better to be straightforward and use positive terms in your sentence. For example, the advertising slogan *Don't let Australia down* is a double negative that would be more positively phrased as *Take Australia forward*. A politician recently said in a radio interview, *I am not ready to disagree with that*, which is poli-speak for *I agree*. Although advertisers may regret the loss of alliteration and politicians the loss of air space, these types of negative constructs have no place in scientific writing. After all, who can make any sense of writing that says *Diet was not a risk factor for asthma in adults but was not in children.*

The meanings of sentences often become clearer when negative words are omitted. For example, writing that *We did not find a statistical interaction between the outcome and exposure variables* could suggest that you did not even look for one. Rather, it is clearer to write that *There was no significant interaction between the outcome and exposure variable (P = 0·91).* The direct expression and the inclusion of the *P* value shows that you tested for an interaction and found that it was statistically non-significant.

Similarly, try not to use negative sentence constructions such as *We did not find that weight loss was related to age* that suggest that you may not have tested for a relation. It is much better to say that *There was no relation between age and weight loss*, which describes exactly what you mean. In the same vein, phrases such as *We found no evidence that* are often better rephrased with *We did not find any evidence that.* No one can find nothing, although you can demonstrate that something is not present.

Box 10.5 Switching from negative to positive

1 ✘ Two patients were excluded from the intention-to-treat analysis because they <u>received no study drugs</u>
  ✓ Two patients were excluded from the intention-to-treat analysis because they did not receive the allocated treatment

2 ✘ <u>No mechanism</u> was observed between airborne fungal concentrations and emergency department attendance
  ✓ Emergency department attendance was not related to airborne fungal concentrations

3 ✘ While the majority of cases onset in the first two weeks of life, later onset is <u>not unknown</u>
  ✓ The majority of cases have their onset in the first two weeks of life but later onset sometimes occurs
  ✓ In the majority of cases, the disease is evident in the first two weeks although some cases are not diagnosed until later in life

4 ✘ This drug will <u>not only be invaluable</u> in the treatment of children but <u>may be</u> valuable in adults also
  ✓ This drug will be valuable in the treatment of children and may be valuable in adults also
  ✓ This drug is effective for treating children and may also be effective in adults

5 ✖ A single outcome measurement <u>will often be inadequate</u> to assess the risks, costs and diverse benefits that may arise from the use of a new treatment

✓ The diverse benefits that may result from the use of a new treatment can rarely be measured by a single outcome variable

6 ✖ Authors of published abstracts were significantly <u>less likely</u> to believe that a journal <u>would not publish</u> their manuscript than authors of rejected abstracts

✓ Authors of published abstracts were significantly more likely to believe that a journal would publish their manuscript than authors of rejected abstracts

Some examples of unclear uses of negatives are shown in Box 10.5. In the first example, patients cannot receive *nothing* and, in the second example, you cannot observe *no mechanism*. Both sentences benefit from being rewritten to remove the inappropriate negative and express a more exact meaning. Example 3 shows a typical double negative phrase. In this example, which was used to describe the recognition of a genetic disease, the term *onset* was also inappropriate. Genes do not change over time, although it may be a while before the identifying symptoms are recognised. The sentence needs to reflect this even if extra words are needed.

In the fourth example, the double negative is better removed and the word *valuable* exchanged for a more specific and unambiguous term. This sentence does not work well because the two phrases that include the stem word *valuable* are constructed in a non-parallel way. In addition, the terms *valuable* and *invaluable* may mean different things to different people, whereas the term *effective* has a precise scientific meaning. In examples 5 and 6, the use of negatives is unnecessary and the sentences are better phrased using positive words.

Abbreviations

A place for everything, and everything in its place.

Samuel Smith (1812–1904)

Abbreviations should also be avoided whenever possible. Unless your abbreviation refers to a standard measurement,

Table 10.2 Standard and non-standard abbreviations.	
Standard abbreviations: define and use	**Non-standard abbreviations: do not use**
DNA (deoxyribose nucleic acid)	DD (doubling dose)
ECG (electrocardiogram)	PAR (perennial allergic rhinitis)
IgE (immunoglobulin E)	FUO (fever of unknown origin)
SIDS (sudden infant death syndrome)	OPT (optic pathway tumour)
BMI (body mass index)	TAI (total allergy index)
FVC (forced vital capacity)	VPI (very preterm infants)

such as cm or mm, the full term for which it stands should precede its first use in the text. Once an abbreviation is defined, then you must use it throughout your paper in preference to the full expression.

The uniform requirements for manuscripts[5] states that only standard abbreviations should be used in the text and that abbreviations should not be used at all in the abstract and in the title (www[2]). This is excellent advice. It is certainly not a good idea to invent your own abbreviations that the reader has to remember while reading your paper. It is even harder for readers when you invent two or three new abbreviations and use them throughout the paper. This practice of creating alphabet soup detracts from clarity and readability. Table 10.2 shows some standard and non-standard abbreviations.

Spelling

> *Why is the word dictionary in the dictionary and if it was misspelled, how would we know? Where did Webster look up the definitions when he wrote the dictionary? Why can't you make another word using all the letters in "anagram".*

> Taken from an internet bulletin board

Poor spelling must be avoided at all costs because it annoys readers, can be confusing if another meaning is attached to a word and, with the advent of computer programs with dictionaries and spell-checking facilities, is no longer excusable. Although some sympathy is often extended to researchers who have to write in English rather than their own language, most reviewers find incorrect spelling irritating. If you know that you are prone to spelling a word incorrectly, then you should search your paper for that word and replace it correctly.

Be aware that the spell checker may not pick up an incorrectly spelt word if the form you have used is a valid sequence of letters. For example, you may type *you* instead of *your* or *rates* instead of *rats*. There is no substitute for careful proofreading, and careful peer reviewers and copy editors. You will also have to choose a spelling standard that is appropriate for the journal that you send your paper to. Some journals are quite specific about which dictionary to use, for example the *BMJ* recommends *Chambers 21st century dictionary* for general use and *Dorlands dictionary* for medical terms and the *Australia and New Zealand Journal of Psychiatry* requests that papers are spell-checked using the *Macquarie dictionary*.

One hitch with spelling is that the Americans and English spell some words differently. For example, Americans use *z* instead of *s* in words such as *minimise* and *organise*, and drop the *a* from words such as *aetiology* and *paediatrics* and the *o* from words like *oestrogen*. They also write *mold* not *mould*. The differences are endless. You have two choices. Either spell consistently in American or spell consistently in English but do not chop and change between the two. Most word-processing programs allow you to choose whether you want to use an American or English dictionary to spell check your work.

Words matter

> *Parameter. Use this nasty vogue word and I'll forgive you only if you're a mathematician, a scientist, or a computer programmer. (Even then, I'll probably forgive you only grudgingly.) The rest of the world can safely do without.*
>
> Jack Lynch (www[1])

The words that you choose and the ways in which you use them are the crux of good writing. The tricks that will help you to become an expert wordsmith are shown in Box 10.6.

> ## Box 10.6 Word tips
>
> Standardise all terms
> Maintain consistency in orders and viewpoints
> Check that the words mean what you want them to mean
> Adhere to humanising and non-emotive terms
> Avoid double or unnecessary negatives
> Only use standard abbreviations
> Spell check and proofread your paper

Acknowledgements

The Smith quote has been produced with permission from *Collins Concise Dictionary of Quotations, 3rd edn*. London: Harper Collins, 1998 (p 299). the Lederman quote has been produced with permission from Horvitz, LA ed. *The Quotable Scientist*. New York: McGraw-Hill Companies, 2000 (p 23). The Orwell quote has been produced with permission from the Orwell estate (Secker and Warburg). All other referenced quotes have been produced with permission.

Websites

1 The Writing Program, University of Pennsylvania
   http://www.sas.upenn.edu/writing/services/docs.html
   Access to online reference texts and resources including *Grammar style and notes* by Jack Lynch, *Strunk's elements of style, Oxford English Dictionary, Webster's dictionary, Roget's thesaurus*, citation styles, etc.

2 International Committee of Medical Journal Editors (ICMJE)
   http://www.icmje.org
   Uniform requirements that provide instructions to authors on how to prepare manuscripts to submit to biomedical journals, including links to sites about sponsorship, authorship, and accountability

References

1 Dunn I. *The writer's guide*. Sydney: Allen and Unwin, 1999; p 5.
2 Zeiger M. *Essentials of writing biomedical research papers*. Maidenhead: McGraw-Hill, 1991; p 2.
3 Boynton PM. People should participate in, not be subjects of, research. *BMJ* 1998;**317**:1521.
4 Aronson J. When I use a word. Now concentrate. *BMJ* 1999;**319**:494.
5 International Committee of Medical Journal Editors. Uniform requirements for manuscripts submitted to biomedical journals. *Ann Intern Med* 1997;**126**:36–47.

11: Punctuation

More people fear snakes than fear full stops, which could explain why they recoil when a long sentence comes hissing across the page.

Martin Cutts[1]

The objectives of this chapter are to understand how to:

- choose the correct punctuation
- avoid incorrect commas and apostrophes
- write correctly punctuated sentences

Full stops and ellipses

The great saxophonist John Coltrane was troubled because his solos were running way too long. He couldn't figure out how to end his improvisations. His friend Miles Davies had a suggestion. "John" he said, "put the horn down."

Patricia O'Conner[2]

The use of a full stop is simple – it shows where the sentence ends. If you are writing short, snappy sentences, the full stop will be by far the most common punctuation mark that you will ever use. Occasionally, full stops are replaced by exclamation marks or by question marks. Because all three punctuation marks fulfil the same role of ending the sentence, only one is used at a time.

The rules for using full stops are not so much when to use them as when not to use them. Full stops are not needed after titles, in people's names, in abbreviations or acronyms. Full stops can certainly be omitted from the following: *Dr D Brown, DNA, 7 am, 160 cm,* etc.

Ellipses are a series of full stops that are used to indicate the omission of quoted text. For example, in the sentence *The patient had a stroke ... but after many months of treatment ... returned to work*, the ellipses replace omitted text. Such constructions would rarely be used in a journal article but may be used for quotations in reviews, letters, and other documents.

Question and exclamation marks

> *Anyone who wishes to become a good writer should endeavour, before he allows himself to be tempted by the more showy qualities, to be direct, simple, brief, vigorous, and lucid.*
>
> HW Fowler
> (www.bartelby.com)

Naturally enough, question marks are used to end a sentence that asks a direct question such as *What is the patient's diagnosis?* However, a question mark is not used to end indirect questions such as *The patients were asked how they felt.*

An exclamation mark is used to indicate surprise and is almost never used in the non-emotive world of scientific writing. Because question marks and exclamations replace a full stop, they are never followed by a full stop.

Colons and semicolons

> *Experience is a wonderful thing. It enables you to recognise a mistake when you make it.*
>
> Taken from an internet bulletin board

In scientific writing, colons are rarely used in the text. The main purpose of using a colon is to introduce a list, as for example in *We collected data from the following four centres: Lismore, Belmont, Sydney, and Broken Hill.* However, colons are sometimes used in a title to introduce the study design or setting without introducing a full stop.[3] The wisdom of this is discussed in Chapter 4.

Semicolons are used even less often than colons. Semicolons are a watered down full stop but are stronger than a comma and, as such, command a longer pause in thought. In practice, it is usually better to use a full stop and delineate ideas into sentences rather than use semicolons that tend to perpetuate long, snaky sentences.

Commas

> *Be sparing with commas. Putting them in every few words prevents the reader from getting the construction of the sentence.*
>
> Martin Cutts[1]

Commas are used to separate parts of a sentence that can't run together. Commas give readers a time to pause and take in the meanings of the words. The words between two commas in a sentence, between a comma and the full stop, or at the beginning of a sentence before a comma, cordon off information that is additional to the main message of the sentence and that is therefore non-essential.

It is important not to overuse commas and never to use a comma in place of a full stop. It is not a good idea to use "comma splices", that is a comma to join together two separate sentences. Such run on sentences are ungrammatical. Either use two short sentences or join the sentences together with a conjunction rather than a comma.

Commas are also used to separate adjectives when they appear as a list before a noun, for example *small, unrepresentative samples of women*. However, commas are not used in word clusters to describe a disease or in word clusters that form a proper noun, for example *non-insulin dependent diabetes* or *National Nutrition Survey* (see Box 3.2 in Chapter 3).

Some sentences in which commas are correctly used and some situations in which commas should not be used are shown in Table 11.1. Examples 1–6 show the correct uses of commas. One rule is to never use a comma after *but, and,* or *or*

Table 11.1 When, and when not to, use a comma.

		Examples
When to use a comma		
1	When a sentence begins with a conjunction	However, we will need to order some new equipment
2	When a sentence begins with an essential or non-essential dependent clause	Before the study begins, we will need to order some new equipment We will need to order some new equipment before the study begins
3	When a non-essential adjectival clause is embedded into an independent clause or ends a sentence	The equipment, which we can order from the university supplier, will be needed before the study begins We will need to buy some new equipment, which we can order from the university supplier
4	When two phrases with the same meaning are used side by side	Professor Brown, the vice chancellor, will attend the meeting
5	To separate items in a list (American English adds a comma before the final "and" and this positioning helps to avoid ambiguity)	Questionnaires will be used to measure demography, age, gender, and illness history
6	To avoid ambiguity	When the final speaker finishes, the keynote address will begin
When not to use a comma		
7	When the independent clause starts a sentence and is followed by an essential dependent clause	✗ We shall need to buy new equipment, that can be used to measure ambient humidity ✓ We shall need to buy new equipment that can be used to measure ambient humidity
8	When the independent clause is embedded with an essential, dependent clause	✗ The new equipment that we shall need, can be ordered from the university supplier ✓ The new equipment that we shall need can be ordered from the university supplier
9	To separate two independent clauses	✗ Many existing tools have been criticised for poor validity, furthermore, most are based on a single measurement ✓ Many existing tools have been criticised for poor validity. Furthermore, most are based on a single measurement

when this word occurs mid-sentence. In examples 7–9, the commas need to be deleted.

Commas are not used in dates. Dates are written as 4 January 2002 with no comma before the year. Box 11.1 shows some examples in which commas have been used incorrectly and that are corrected simply by repairing the punctuation.

Box 11.1 Putting commas in the right places

1 ✗ After six days surviving colonies were counted, and expressed as a percentage of the number of colonies in the control group
   ✓ After six days, surviving colonies were counted and the number was expressed as a percentage of the number of colonies in the control group

2 ✗ For some diseases immunity, from infection and/or vaccination, may wane with time
   ✓ For some diseases, immunity induced by infection or vaccination may decrease with time

3 ✗ At four of the hospitals the research nurses placed screening questionnaires, in the medical records of people attending the clinic
   ✓ At four of the hospitals, the research nurses placed screening questionnaires in the medical records of potential participants

4 ✗ The therapeutic gene and the "advantage" gene would be delivered, to the liver, together in a single vector
   ✓ The therapeutic gene and the "advantage" gene would be delivered to the liver in a single vector

5 ✗ Provided that any biases remain reasonably constant over time the screening method may be used for monitoring of shifts in effectiveness over time, rather than for precise point estimates
   ✓ Provided that any bias remains reasonably constant, this screening method can be used for monitoring changes in effectiveness over time rather than for obtaining point estimates

6 ✗ The concept of self-management, which has at its core, an increase in patient autonomy is problematic
   ✓ The concept of self-management, which is based on patient autonomy, is problematic

7 ✗ Although we believe, or feel comfortable with the notion, that all patients want to control their own management many patients are reluctant to make their own treatment choices

(continued)

> ✓ Although many practitioners are comfortable with the notion of patients controlling their own management, many patients are reluctant to make their own treatment choices
>
> 8 ✘ A total of 241 patients were seen at the clinic between November, 1999 and January, 2000
> ✓ A total of 241 patients were seen at the clinic between November 1999 and January 2000

One of the quirks of writing is that Americans use commas differently from the English and even the English are not consistent. Some English journals chose to omit the comma after an introductory phrase or clause but others retain commas as a means of cordoning off the phrase and improving readability. The most noticeable international difference is that Americans consistently use commas both between independent clauses and before the final item in a list. A comma before the final item in a list, which is called an "Oxford comma", is used by some English journals also, including the *BMJ*.

As with your choice of spelling, you have two choices. You should write correctly using English or American punctuation depending on the journal to which you want to submit your paper, or you can write entirely in one style and rely on the copy editors of the journal to add or remove extra commas. However, to avoid confusing your readers, you must avoid changing between the two styles within a paper.

Apostrophes

The apostrophe is now so widely misused – an errant tadpole one columnist calls it – that its eventual death seems inevitable. Alongside their no-smoking stickers, companies could soon be declaring themselves apostrophe free zones. This would be a pity, as the correct use of apostrophes conveys meaning and prevents ambiguity, while misplaced apostrophes make the reader stumble and backtrack.

Martin Cutts[1]

It is amazing how often writers see an "s" at the end of a word and feel the need to add an apostrophe. In the following subheading taken from a magazine, both the comma and the apostrophe are used incorrectly: *Advice on a perennial problem, from a top rider who has to cope with horses'*. In this title, both the comma and the final apostrophe should be omitted.

The need for an apostrophe is an exception rather than a rule. Nouns and pronouns only have an apostrophe before the final "s" when they indicate possession. For example, in the sentence *We measured the participant's height* the apostrophe in *participant's* is used to mean *of the* to indicate possession. The other most common use of an apostrophe is when you need to signal that some letters are missing. For example, when *it's* is short for *it is* or *it has*. In the following sentence the apostrophe is correctly used: *When the equipment is overloaded, <u>its</u> instrumentation signals that <u>it's</u> not recording information*.

When an "s" is added to signal a plural noun, an apostrophe is definitely not needed even when it is added to a number. For example, we write *in the 1970s*. The following sentences demonstrate the correct use of apostrophes to indicate possession when writing singular and plural nouns: *Clear writing is easy on the reader's mind* or *Clear paragraphs are easy on readers' minds*.

When a plural noun ends with an "s", an apostrophe is added but the final "s" is omitted. Finally, possessive pronouns do not have an apostrophe so that you write *hers* not *her's*. Is this all too complicated? No, not really. Once you have learnt the rules, which are shown in Table 11.2, you will have them with you forever.

Parentheses and square brackets

Don't bury important ideas in parentheses.

Jack Lynch (www[1])

Parentheses, or round brackets, are used to contain an abbreviation or acronym when it is first explained, for example *In this study, we measured systolic blood pressure (SBP)*.

Table 11.2 Use of apostrophes to indicate possession.

Condition	Examples
For singular or plural nouns that do not end in "s", add an apostrophe and an "s"	The doctor's stethoscope The patient's belongings The children's toys
For plural nouns that end in "s", add an apostrophe	The patients' waiting room
For singular nouns that end in "s", add an apostrophe and an "s" (with the exception of a few words such as Jesus', Moses' where last syllable is pronouned)	Dr Barnes's paper
For phrases, add the apostrophe and an "s" to the last word	The Chief of Staff's book
For joint ownership, add an apostrophe and an "s" to the last name	Barnes and Smith's paper
When there is no joint ownership, add an apostrophe and an "s" to each name	Smith's and Miller's papers
Pronouns that are already possessive do not need apostrophes	His, hers, its, theirs, yours

Once an abbreviation is explained, you must use the term in its abbreviated form throughout your paper. If you are only using a term occasionally, it should always be used in full. It is not worth creating alphabet soup by using abbreviations that have to be remembered but that are only used once or twice.

Parentheses are also used to cordon off a group of words that add an explanation to the sentence but that are relatively unimportant. Parentheses are used to enclose text that adds non-essential details to clarify a point. Because scientific writing has no place for unimportant asides, parentheses are usually used only for definitions and abbreviations. In the following sentences, parentheses are correctly used to define the size of the study centres and to contain the abbreviations:

The rural towns chosen were Wagga Wagga (population 40 000) and Belmont (population 20 000) or *In this study, we measured the prevalence of airway hyperresponsiveness (AHR), recent wheeze*

(wheeze in the 12 months prior to study) and atopy (a positive skin prick test to one or more inhaled allergens).

Parentheses cannot be used to cordon off large phrases or clauses that contain a verb. Some examples of how to avoid using parentheses are shown in Box 11.2.

Box 11.2 Removing brackets

1 ✖ Flow rates may be decreased for a number of different physiological reasons including loss of elastic recoil, large airways narrowing (as with smooth muscle contraction in asthma) and small airway narrowing (due to a small number of pathological processes including inflammation and changes in small muscle tone)

 ✓ Flow rates may be limited for a number of different physiological reasons – including loss of elastic recoil, large airway narrowing as a result of smooth muscle contraction, and small airway narrowing as a result of pathological processes, such as inflammation and changes in small muscle tone

2 ✖ The occurrence of thunderstorms was not associated with a significant risk of an epidemic of asthma (although it is acknowledged that the confidence interval around the estimate is broad)

 ✓ The occurrence of thunderstorms was not a significant risk factor for an epidemic of asthma, although there was a wide confidence interval around the estimate

3 ✖ Information was available for over 35 070 patient encounters (usually visits) resulting in 61 445 diagnostic contacts (patients can have more than one diagnosis) for the six years, 1978–1982 and 1985

 ✓ For the six years 1978–1982 and 1985, information was available for over 35 070 patient encounters, which were usually doctor visits. Because many patients had more than one diagnosis, there were 61 445 diagnostic contacts

---

Square brackets are rarely used in scientific writing. Occasionally, they may be used to include words or phrases that are added by someone other than the author of the text. For example, a copy editor may add information as follows: *The pilot study was carried out in Newcastle [Australia] and the results show that there has been a significant decrease in infant mortality [turn to p. 46].*

Slashes, dashes, and hyphens

Slashes are far too common and almost always betray a lazy thinker.

Jack Lynch (www[1])

A slash is often used when two words are related and the writer does not know how they are related, or when two words can be used alternatively. In most cases, a slash can be replaced by the word *or*. For example, in the sentence *We need to measure whether the prevalence of this illness has increased/ decreased in the last five years*, the slash could be replaced by *or*, or the cluster *increased/decreased* could be replaced by *changed*.

Dashes and hyphens are described in the language of typographers as the em rule, the two-em rule and the en rule. A dash is known as an "em rule" because it is the width of an "m" and a long dash is known as a "two-em rule" because it is twice as long. The "en rule" is shorter or about half the length of an em rule. The "spaced en rule" is an en rule with a space either side.

An em rule or a dash, which is a long hyphen, is another punctuation mark that is rarely used in scientific writing. A dash is usually used to replace a parenthesis or to interrupt the flow of text. For example, in the sentence *Flow rates may be limited for many physiological reasons—including loss of elastic recoil—which need to be examined,* the dashes are used to replace commas. In this sentence, commas would be preferable. However, if you use dashes the copy editor may decide to replace them with commas or to use a spaced en rule, whichever is the publisher's house style.

The en rule is a short dash used to join words or to mean *to* when joining numbers, for example as in *1972–1992* or *May–July*.

As with all punctuation, try to be minimal in your use of hyphens. Hyphens can be used safely when a word begins with '*non-*' such as *non-essential, non-clinical*, etc. Hyphens are also used for words that include a preposition, such as *run-in phase*, and to create noun clusters such as *self-management*, although they are often omitted, for example in words such as *outlier* rather than '*out-lier.*' Many word clusters, such as *risk factor*, *breast feeding* and *birth weight* do not need hyphens and, in some cases, are joined to form a single word. In some journals, there is a trend towards using as few hyphens as possible so that *re-write* is spelt *rewrite*, *pre-school* is spelt *preschool* and *follow-up* is spelt *followup*.

Punctuation matters

> *The notion that a scientific paper should be written in a special language is nonsense. It should be in good, plain English. People do not ambulate and take oral fluids; they walk and they drink.*

> John Ellard[4]

The rules of punctuation are simple and few and add style to your writing. The effort it takes to master the rules will pay huge dividends in giving you confidence in using punctuation correctly. Just knowing when to cordon off words correctly with commas can give a smart look to your writing. Box 11.3 shows the four rules of punctuation that you will need to check out in your writing. Further information can be found at some websites (www[2–3]).

Box 11.3 Checking out the punctuation

End sentences with full stops
Avoid colons and semicolons when possible
Put commas and apostrophes in the correct places
Eliminate all but the most essential hyphens and brackets

Acknowledgements

The O'Conner quotes: excerpts from *Words Fail Me: What Everyone Who Writes Should Know About Writing*, copyright © 1999 by Patricia O'Conner have been reprinted by permission of Harcourt, Inc. All referenced quotes in this chapter have been produced with permission.

Websites

1 The Writing Program, University of Pennsylvania
   http://www.sas.upenn.edu/writing/services/docs.html

Access to online reference texts and resources including *Grammar style and notes* by Jack Lynch, *Strunk's elements of Style, Oxford English Dictionary, Webster's dictionary, Roget's thesaurus*, citation styles, etc.

2 Modern Language Association (MLA) of America
http://www.mla.org
http://www.mla.org/main_stl.htm#sources
Information about the *MLA style manual* which documents the style recommended by the Modern Language Association for preparing scholarly manuscripts and student research papers. This website provides information about the mechanics of writing, such as punctuation, quotation, and documentation of sources. Also includes guidelines for citing sources from the World Wide Web

3 Plain English Campaign
http://www.plainenglish.co.uk
Guides to writing medical information, letters, reports, alternative words, etc. for writing in plain English

References

1 Cutts M. *The plain English guide*. Oxford: Oxford University Press, 1995; pp 11, 85, 89.
2 O'Conner P. *Words fail me*. London: Harcourt, 1999; p 99.
3 Cameron H, Robertson A. The colon in medicine: nothing to do with the intestinal tract. *BMJ* 1997;**315**:1657–8.
4 Ellard J. How to make an editor's life easier. *Australasian Psychiatry* 2001;9:212–14.

12: Support systems

If I have seen further (than certain other men) it is by standing on the shoulders of giants.

Isaac Newton (British physicist, 1642–1727)

The objectives of this chapter are to understand how to:

- find new writing resources
- improve your writing through group learning
- mentor new writers

There are some essential items that every writer needs in their tool box. These include a good dictionary and thesaurus. To this can be added any number of reference books, inspirational articles, or resource materials that provide useful information about writing and grammar (www[1-5]). Also, no one can write a paper by themselves. In addition to the help you will receive from your coauthors, there are other valuable systems, including mentors, writers' groups, and the internet that can provide information and support.

Searching the internet

Je ne cherche pas; je trouve. I do not search; I find.

Pablo Picasso (1881–1973)

The internet has grown in an extraordinary way and offers many scientific and educational sites that may be useful for your research or your writing. However, spending time surfing the internet is not an efficient way to find the materials that are most relevant to your work. The search engine Google™ (www[6]) has over 1·6 million web pages and continues to grow. Surfing sites such as this will waste your time and may never lead you to the best information available. Finding the most appropriate information on the internet depends on using precise queries and using search engines effectively.

For efficient searches, it is important to use precise descriptive terms on a large international search engine such as Google™, Altavista® or All-the-Web® (www[6-8]). By entering specific words in the query box of a search engine, you will retrieve web pages that contain all of the words. Using effective search techniques will narrow your search to a manageable number of results. However, each search engine has a slightly different searching technique. To become a competent searcher, choose a search engine that most suits your needs and become familiar with its search techniques.

Most engines offer different levels from basic to advanced searching. To help with searching, Google™ has a search tip (www[9]) and Altavista® has a search cheat sheet (www[10]). There are many other useful features available through the search engines such as Altavista's babelfish translation tool (www[11]). Because the features of search engines change regularly, it is useful to visit the search help pages to keep up to date with the changes and the features they offer.

There are also a number of websites that offer tutorials that will help you to search more effectively, for example The Spire Project (www[12]) and Bright Planet (www[13]). With efficient searching, the internet can become an essential tool to help you to conduct your research, analyse your data, and publish your results.

Writers' groups

> Let's face it. Writing is hell.
>
> William Styron (US novelist, b. 1925)
> (www.bartelby.com)

So much about science is about getting feedback from peers and this is especially important when it comes to writing. One effective way to elicit feedback and to update your writing skills is to form or join a writers' group. Writers' groups are a good way for researchers to share their experiences of endless drafts, the acceptance or rejection of a paper and bad writing days. They are also a good way to share successes and to receive support, encouragement, and affirmation from colleagues.

In most research teams, some people will have been writing for a long time and others will be beginners. A writers' group is an excellent way for juniors to pick up writing skills from seniors and for seniors to be kept up to speed by their junior colleagues. Such groups are especially important for postgraduate and postdoctoral students who need to build up their research experience and their scientific writing skills. Writers' groups can foster self-motivation, clear thinking, and an appreciation of team approaches. They can also help writers to set realistic time-lines, choose the right style in which to present their work and fast track their publication rates.

For senior researchers, having a formal venue in which to help junior colleagues makes them better researchers and also makes them better people too. Some researchers, no matter how junior or senior, like to work on other people's writing as a way of improving their own writing skills. Brave souls are happy to ask for feedback on their own writing from a group of fellow researchers who will be honest and helpful. It takes great courage to ask for your work to be reviewed in public – this has been likened to putting your head in the lion's mouth![1] You have to have a certain fortitude to be able to accept criticism in front of your peers. However, such criticism is valuable for reducing the number of drafts that you need to write and for pushing a paper along the path to being published.

Box 12.1 Organising a writers' group

We are planning to conduct a writers' group for researchers who are in the process of preparing journal articles for publication. The purpose of this group is to provide a regular, interactive forum in which participants can learn the skills of writing and reviewing scientific articles.

The meetings will include some teaching about how to construct a paper and the rules of grammar but will be mostly interactive. At each meeting, we will review some examples of writing that will include participants' own manuscripts where possible. The group will be limited to a small number of participants who should plan to attend regularly. Meetings will be held on the first Tuesday of each month.

Box 12.1 shows an example of how to advertise for writers to join the group. People in the group should be prepared to review other writers' work and make suggestions, give positive feedback, and reiterate writing rules.

Groups of four to six writers who meet once a month or every second week work well. Bigger groups of more than eight writers should probably be split into two to work effectively. Meeting regularly gives everyone a date to commit to and an informal deadline for preparing or reviewing work in progress. The time between meetings must be long enough so that writers have time to take on board suggestions and revise their work. A large meeting space is not necessary but good coffee or appealing snacks work well. Above all else, writers' groups provide a venue to talk productively about publishing and to share skills that improve writing. These meetings can be a lot of fun too.

If researchers are both brave and willing, they can bring along pieces of their writing for others to comment on. Even better, once the writing is revised, bringing along the final product can inspire others to use the same approach. However, if some of the people are not confident enough to bring along their own writing, you can begin by using papers from the literature and discussing how you would have put them together. It is polite though, to choose papers from a different city or country. No researcher would want their work to be criticised by a group meeting at the end of their corridor.

In any learning group, it is good to have a facilitator who can set some ground rules. It is important to be gentle when reviewing anyone's work. In writing comments on someone's paper, it is best to use pencil because this looks more like suggestions than criticisms written in ink. Red ink is especially seen as a loud command. Of course, pencil comments do not transmit well by fax and may not be readable under poor lighting conditions. As a reviewer, it is always important to consider how to give feedback that will be accepted as a positive path to better writing and that will encourage productivity.

Writers must also be sensitive in the way in which they give verbal feedback. Above all, group members must be honest and encouraging without being rude, abrupt, or dismissive.

They need to use gentle communication skills such as saying *The reader may be confused here* rather than *This section confuses me* or *I can't understand what this means*. A good review skill is to congratulate writers on parts of their work that you like before highlighting any poor writing or lack of clarity that you find. It sometimes works well if the reviewer explains the problem but lets the writer find a solution to fix it. Reviewers should be clear that writing always belongs to the writer whose job it is to decide whether or not to accept or reject any suggestions.

Reviewers are, by definition, people who commit their time to read a document and who endeavour to make helpful suggestions. In return for being treated with respect, writers should accept review comments gracefully. It is not a good idea to go into battle with reviewers about who is right or wrong. There are no rights and wrongs in scientific writing – it is all a matter of preference and balance.

Once you have formed a writers' group, you will need to create your own mini-lessons that will be directed by what the group is interested in learning. Whatever the exercises, it is important that the content material is appropriate for the people in the group. If the writers are all from a specialised research area, it is most appropriate to use examples from that discipline. However, if the writers are from mixed research areas, then writing on general topics that are easily understood by everyone should be used. Box 12.2 shows some activities that writers' groups can consider using.

Box 12.2 Writers' group activities

Collect examples of good writing
Circulate any inspiring, motivating, or educational materials
Review writing in progress
Hold 2-minute writing clinics
Reduce abstracts or letters by 20%
Have fun word spotting
Share ideas about improving writing productivity
Run a workshop on time-management strategies

Writers can collect examples of good writing that they share with the group and any resource materials that they discover.

Members of the group can bring along any inspirational material that they find. They can also bring examples of writing that the group can review. If writers can bring a tortuous title or a couple of foggy sentences that they have spotted in the journals or media, a 2-minute writing clinic to put things right is very satisfying. Examples of 2-minute writing clinics to rewrite titles are shown in Box 12.3. In the first example, the word *training* is used twice and is a sure indication that the title could be shortened. The second title can also be made much briefer.

Box 12.3 Examples of 2-minute clinics for rewriting titles

1 ✖ Risk factors for training-related injuries among men and women in basic sports training
  ✓ Risk factors for injury during basic sports training

2 ✖ Long-term risk of second malignancy in survivors of acute lymphoblastic leukaemia treated during adolescence or young adulthood
  ✓ Long-term outcomes in young survivors of acute lymphoblastic leukaemia
  ✓ Risk of second malignancy in young survivors of acute lymphoblastic leukaemia

---

In addition to titles, examples of foggy writing to use in 2-minute writing clinics can be found from many sources as shown in Box 12.4. Example 1 came from an in-flight magazine, example 2 from a letter to hospital staff, example 3 from the instructions on a pack of an over-the-counter medication, and example 4 from a departmental email. To remedy this type of writing, it is just a matter of writing tightly and writing clearly. Neither the long nor the short version is right or wrong but the short versions are more readable. They are also more easily understood, which is what we want for scientific writing. In writers' groups, you will discover that there may be several correct ways to write each sentence and choosing which one is best is often a matter of personal preference.

Box 12.4 Examples of 2-minute clinics for rewriting text

1 ✱ During long flights individuals are at risk of deep venous thrombosis and should ambulate regularly and ensure adequate oral fluid because immmobility and dehydration have been implicated in the aetiology of deep venous thrombosis
   ✓ Regular exercise and frequent drinks of water will decrease the risk of blood clots forming in your leg veins during long flights

2 ✱ The administration acknowledges that car parking for staff at the Children's Hospital is currently very limited and in this respect an action plan is currently being developed with a view to alleviating the problems
   ✓ We realise that car parking at the hospital is very limited and we are planning to improve the situation

3 ✱ Alleviates the discomfort associated with internal and external haemorrhoids, pruritis ani and other related anorectal conditions. Apply night and morning and after each evacuation. Children: no dose recommended
   ✓ Relieves pain and itchiness around the anus caused by piles. Use in the morning, at night, and after emptying your bowel. Not recommended for children

4 ✱ Before deciding on a proposed location for the new laboratories, we will need to conduct further investigations into the safety issues involved and make an economic assessment of the advantages and disadvantages of the various sites available
   ✓ Before finalising a location for the new laboratories, we will investigate the safety issues and economic advantages of the proposed sites

One exercise is to take any abstract from a paper on MEDLINE® (www[14]) or any letter in a journal and reduce the word count by 20% without deleting any important information. Such exercises, which take only 10 minutes or so, demonstrate how many excess words are used in published writing and how much clearer the text becomes without them.

It is also good fun to spend some time word spotting. One week underline all the nouns in a paragraph and then identify the adjectives and discuss whether they add or detract from the clarity of the text. At other meetings, do the verbs and adverbs, nouns and pronouns, prepositions and conjunctions, etc. These exercises will improve your grammar skills, and identify the parts of sentences and the types of sentence constructions that lead to writing problems.

Writers' groups can also share ideas about how to create writing time and use it productively. You may like to spend some time discussing how to manage "time thieves". Ask everyone in the group to list the tasks that occupy their average working week and divide them into the four quadrants shown in Table 1.1 in Chapter 1. It is prudent to realise that every half-hour spent doing something unimportant can be converted to writing time. Dealing with email is a common time thief but minimising this daily task is simple as shown in Box 12.5. You can also devise lists of how to manage other unimportant activities, for example by delegating work, limiting committee attendance, grouping tasks more efficiently, etc. All of these are good ways to "make time".

Box 12.5 Keeping email under control

❑ Check your email only once or twice a day at specific times and do not spend more than 20 minutes reading emails and replying to them

❑ Select only the important messages to read immediately, delete the unimportant ones and organise a limited number to deal with later

❑ Disable the alert that flashes on your screen each time a new email arrives

❑ Filter personal emails into a different folder from group emails so that you can prioritise how you deal with them

❑ Remove your name from distribution lists that send you many messages that you don't want or hardly ever read

❑ Do not save or file messages that you will never read

Some teams find it very productive to conduct mini-writers groups when the coauthors of a paper meet to discuss data analyses and construct sections of the paper they are writing. This approach requires a close working relationship between coauthors and a commitment to meet regularly to review and revise the paper. If it is possible for coauthors to work in this way, a paper can be fast tracked because problems are sorted out quickly, interactively, and collaboratively. However, meetings such as this still require that one person has the responsibility of being the author and that the coauthors recognise that their role is to make an intellectual contribution and to provide support as a reviewer.

Avoiding writer's block

Create a 'To-Don't' list that contains tasks, rituals, and meetings that you should never waste your time on again. Then stick to it.

Tom Peters (Sydney Morning Herald)

A surprising number of people have 'writer's block' even though they may not admit it. Such people keep themselves busy using diversionary activities so that they can put off writing. It is good to discuss ideas in a workshop about how to combat such activities because there are many tried and tested remedies as shown in Box 12.6. To manage writer's block, you need to be able to recognise it and deal with it. To start with, try taking a few moments to sit at the computer, close your eyes, relax, and get the cricks out of your neck. This will help you to focus on the task and feel relaxed about it. However, you have to get yourself to the computer first. If you are having problems, you need to have some tricks up your sleeve that can be used in times of need.

Box 12.6 Managing writer's block

Learn to recognise the signs and react to them
Join a writers' group and hold a brainstorming session or stress-relieving activities
Seek help from your mentor or supervisor
Take time out to let your brain debrief
Look after your health, diet, and sleep patterns
Have a life outside research with your family and friends
Find inspiration in non-scientific activities (music, art, sport, etc.)
Find a stress-release activity (exercise, walking the dog, movies, etc.)

Ensuring that you quarantine specific time for writing and that you find skills to overcome writer's block are the only ways to make your writing happen. Developing good writing skills makes writing more enjoyable because you can use your time more productively and you will not have to endure endless negative feedback on your draft papers.

Mentoring

A mentor is a kind of career therapist. They are there to see their charges through the ups and downs of their work and help point them in the right direction when they get lost.

Karin Bishop (Sydney Morning Herald, 24 April 1999)

Mentoring happens when a senior researcher shares his or her expertise with a junior researcher. This method of passing on corporate experience to younger colleagues in a trusting way has been used widely over hundreds of years.[2] The first mention of mentoring is in Homer's myth of Odysseus in which Ulysses, the King of Ithaca, entrusts his son to a mentor Telemachus who instructed him for many years whilst Ulysses was fighting the Trojans.[3] With such a well-tried and tested learning method available, it seems a shame not to use it.

Mentors come in many varieties and from many different sources. In research teams, a mentor is often a senior researcher who finds it rewarding to provide advice, support, and encouragement to junior researchers.[3,4] Mentoring is an essential skill for team managers. The most successful researcher team leaders are people who can mentor their students and their junior research staff. The responsibilities that mentors may take on board are summarised in Box 12.7.

Box 12.7 Responsibilities of mentors

Provide advice and support
Impart knowledge, information, guidance, wisdom, and insight
Provide access to research and financial resources
Foster quality and integrity in scientific practice
Promote excellence in scientific writing by reviewing writing regularly and providing timely feedback

---

Provide psychological, social, and emotional encouragement
Motivate and inspire
Provide advice and foster career development
Organise celebrations of important achievements and successes

Because senior researchers can use their corporate experience to contribute to the development of the next generation of scientists, being a mentor can be one of the most rewarding and noble aspects of the research process. The most effective mentors gain satisfaction from helping junior colleagues to conduct research successfully and from guiding inexperienced writers through the writing, review, and publication processes. Good mentors give priority to teaching and learning, agree on objectives, appreciate differences, and find rewards in seeing junior researchers move beyond the realms of their experience. The characteristics of a successful mentor are shown in Box 12.8.

Box 12.8 Characteristics of successful mentors

Encourage excellence in research and scientific writing
Focus on learning and passing on experience
Promote recruitment to higher positions
Provide introductions to new colleagues and networks
Allow for independent development
Help in times of stress or conflict
Have your best interests at heart
Are delighted by your successes

For researchers, a mentor should be a familiar face to turn to in times of stress and a friendly person to rely on when you get stuck. They should provide short-term advice to solve problems and long-term guidance for careers. A mentor should also be a coach who provides pep-talks and is always focused on the goal.[5] As a researcher or scientific writer, you should delight in having a mentor to emulate. Your mentor should allow you to make mistakes in a safe environment while sharing their experiences in helping you to develop your career. We all have our own strengths and weaknesses but to be successful we must build on the strengths and work on the weaknesses. This is where mentors can provide insights in helping researchers to understand the areas that they need to improve and how to improve them. Mentoring is important for teaching writing skills because these can only develop through interactive feedback. By providing positive feedback and constructive criticism, a mentor can help you to become a good writer.[2]

A mentor will also help to increase your self-esteem and self-confidence. Most successful researchers have had at least one mentor to whom they attribute some credit for their progress. If you can find someone to teach you politically savvy ways to become successful, you are much more likely to have a rewarding research career. In recognition of this, professional organisations often have schemes to match junior researchers with a mentor, and web schemes for meeting up with other researchers or for building team work can be found on the internet (www[15–17]).

Parties can meet by email or phone, but regular face-to-face contact to discuss and clarify ideas is essential.[6] Building a relationship with a mentor requires a high level of commitment and honesty on both sides. There is no loss of identity in a healthy mentoring partnership or sense of control on the part of the mentor. When you find a mentor, you will need to work together to set realistic goals and expectations, to decide how frequently to meet and to agree on how your performance will be evaluated. This will enable you to achieve goals that you may have thought were beyond your reach. Box 12.9 lists some of the benefits of mentoring to both mentors and their research units.

Box 12.9 Benefits of mentoring

Enhances teaching and leadership skills
Creates a legacy
Provides exposure to new literature and new research questions
Facilitates coauthorship on journal articles and reviews
Widens the professional network of colleagues and contacts
Increases leadership and job satisfaction
Fosters the development and retention of organisational talent
Contributes to the quality of the scientific profession

The selection of a mentor is an important choice in a research career. If you do not have a mentor in your own research unit, you will need to search further afield. You may find one person to mentor your career path, one to provide research support, and one to help you through the writing and publication processes. If you want a mentor to further your career, you will need someone who is interested in your future. If you want to improve your publication rate, you will need someone who may be a coauthor on your papers, who has an impressive publication record, or who teaches research or scientific writing skills. It doesn't matter how many mentors you have as long as you have all bases covered.

As your career progresses, you will find yourself separating from your mentor. This can be an uncomfortable time but it is part of a natural progression. By then, you will have acquired the skills to successfully mentor those who follow after you. This graduation of junior researchers and sharing of skills and knowledge throughout a research unit can make a huge difference to the success of individual researchers and their research teams.

Acknowledgements

The Newton quote has been produced with permission from *Collins Concise Dictionary of Quotations, 3rd edn*. London: Harper Collins, 1998 (p 226). The Picasso quote has been produced with permission from the Picasso estate (Succession Picasso 2002). All other referenced quotes have been produced with permission.

Websites

1 The Writing Program, University of Pennsylvania
   http://www.sas.upenn.edu/writing/services/docs.html
   Provides access to online reference texts and resources including *Grammar Style* and *Notes* by Jack Lynch, *Strunk's Elements of Style*, *Oxford English Dictionary*, *Webster's Dictionary*, *Roget's Thesaurus*, citation styles, etc.

2 Yahoo
   http://dir.yahoo.com/Social_Science/Linguistics_and_
   Human_Languages/Languages/Specific_Languages/English/
   Grammar__Usage__and_Style/
   Provides access to resources for grammar, English usage, and style, including books and rules of grammar, common errors, and tips to improve your writing

3 Bartelby Online Books
   http://www.bartelby.com
   Access to online books such as the *American Heritage® dictionary, American*

Heritage® book of English usage, Roget's thesaurus, Strunk's elements of style, Gray's anatomy, etc.

4   Modern Language Association (MLA) of America
    http://www.mla.org
    http://www.mla.org/main_stl.htm#sources Information about the MLA style manual, which documents the style recommended by the Modern Language Association for preparing scholarly manuscripts and student research papers. Concerns itself with the mechanics of writing, such as punctuation, quotation, and documentation of sources. Also includes guidelines for citing sources from the World Wide Web

5   Plain English Campaign
    http://www.plainenglish.co.uk
    Guides to writing medical information, letters, reports, alternative words, etc. for writing in plain English

6   Google
    http://www.google.com/
    A unified global search engine

7   Altavista
    http://www.altavista.com/
    A unified global search engine

8   All-the-web, all-the-time
    http://www.alltheweb.com/
    A unified global search engine

9   Google Help Central
    http://www.google.com/help/
    Provides access to a range of search tips, features, and frequently asked questions

10 Altavista's help site
    http://www.altavista.com/sites/help
    Help page with cheat sheets and various searching features

11 Altavista's translation feature
    http://www.altavista.com/sites/help/babelfish/babel_help   Access   to babelfish site that translates from one language to another

12 The Spire Project
    http://www.SpireProject.com/
    Provides access to articles and techniques on internet searching

13 Bright Plant
    http://www.brightplanet.com/
    Provides a guide to effective searching

14 National Library of Medicine, United States
    http://www.nlm.nih.gov/pubs/factsheets/medline.html
    Provides access to abstracts published in MEDLINE® via PubMed®

15 Massachusetts Medical Society
    http://www.globalmedicine.org

Allows health researchers and providers worldwide to establish personal and professional contacts that may lead to cooperative relationships

16 TeamNet, University of North Texas
http://www.workteams.unt.edu/teamnet/teamnet.htm
Electronic community with more than 600 potential mentors who provide a sounding board for ideas and questions

17 Team Center, Washington
http://www.teamcenter.com
Offers articles and tools on effective team building including material on how to ask good questions during meetings, sources of stress in teams, and case studies on teams that work

References

1 Lammott A. *Some instructions on writing and life*. Peterborough: Anchor Books, 1994; p 153.
2 Swap W, Leonard D, Sheilds M, Abrams L. Using mentoring and story telling to transfer knowledge in the workplace. *J Manag Inform Systems* 2001;**18**:95–114.
3 Beech N, Brockbank A. Power/knowledge and psychosocial dynamics in mentoring. *Manag Learning* 1999;**30**:7–24.
4 Gibb S. The usefulness of theory: A case study in evaluating formal mentoring schemes. *Human Relations* 1999;**52**:1055–75.
5 McCabe LL, McCabe ERB. Establishing personal goals and tracking your career. In: *How to succeed in academics*. London: Academic Press, 2000.
6 Daft RL, Lengel RH. Organizational information requirements, media richness and structural design. *Manag Sci* 1986;**32**:554–71.

Index

Page numbers in **bold** type refer to figures; those in *italic* refer to tables or boxed material.